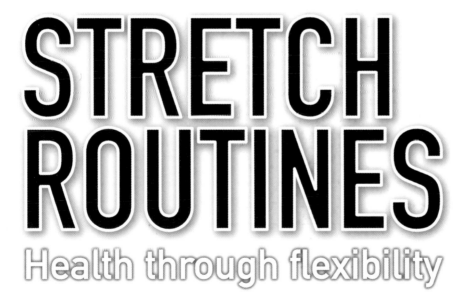

STRETCH ROUTINES
Health through flexibility

Tanya Wyatt

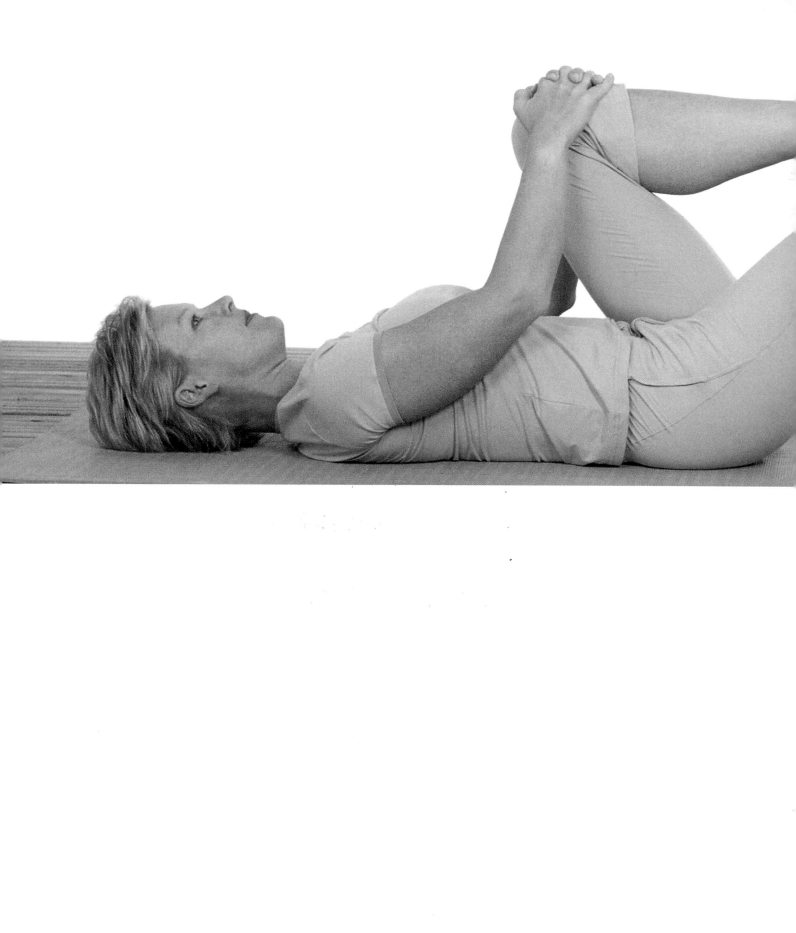

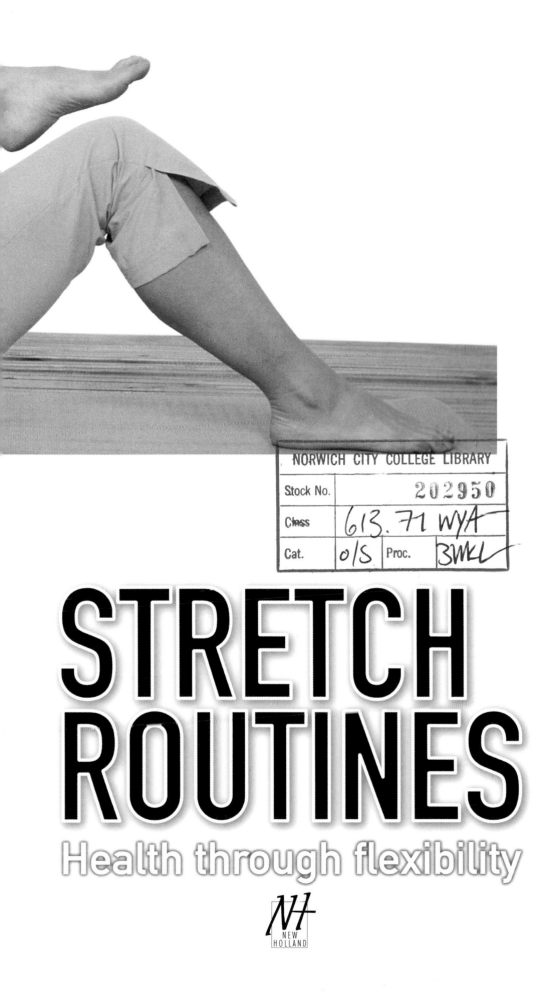

STRETCH ROUTINES

Health through flexibility

NH
NEW
HOLLAND

NEW
HOLLAND

First published in 2004 by New Holland Publishers
London • Cape Town • Sydney • Auckland
www.newhollandpublishers.com

86 Edgware Road, London, W2 2EA, United Kingdom

80 McKenzie Street, Cape Town, 8001, South Africa

14 Aquatic Drive, Frenchs Forest, NSW 2086, Australia

218 Lake Road, Northcote, Auckland, New Zealand

ISBN 1 84330 588 7 (HB)
ISBN 1 84330 589 5 (PB)

Although the publishers have made every effort to ensure that
information contained in this book was meticulously researched
and correct at the time of going to press, they accept no respon-
sibility for any inaccuracies, loss, injury or inconvenience
sustained by any person using this book as reference.

PUBLISHING MANAGERS	Claudia dos Santos & Simon Pooley
COMMISSIONING EDITOR	Alfred LeMaitre
PUBLISHER	Mariëlle Renssen
STUDIO MANAGER	Richard MacArthur
DESIGNER	Geraldine Cupido
DESIGN ASSISTANT	Jeannette Streicher
EDITOR	Anna Tanneberger
ILLUSTRATOR	Steven Felmore
PICTURE RESEARCHER	Karla Kik
PROOFREADER/INDEXER	Michelle Coburn
PRODUCTION	Myrna Collins
CONSULTANT	Dr Nick Walters, Vice Principal British College of Osteopathic Medicine

Reproduction by
Unifoto, Cape Town

Printed and bound in
Singapore by Tien Wah Press (Pte) Ltd

10 9 8 7 6 5 4 3 2 1

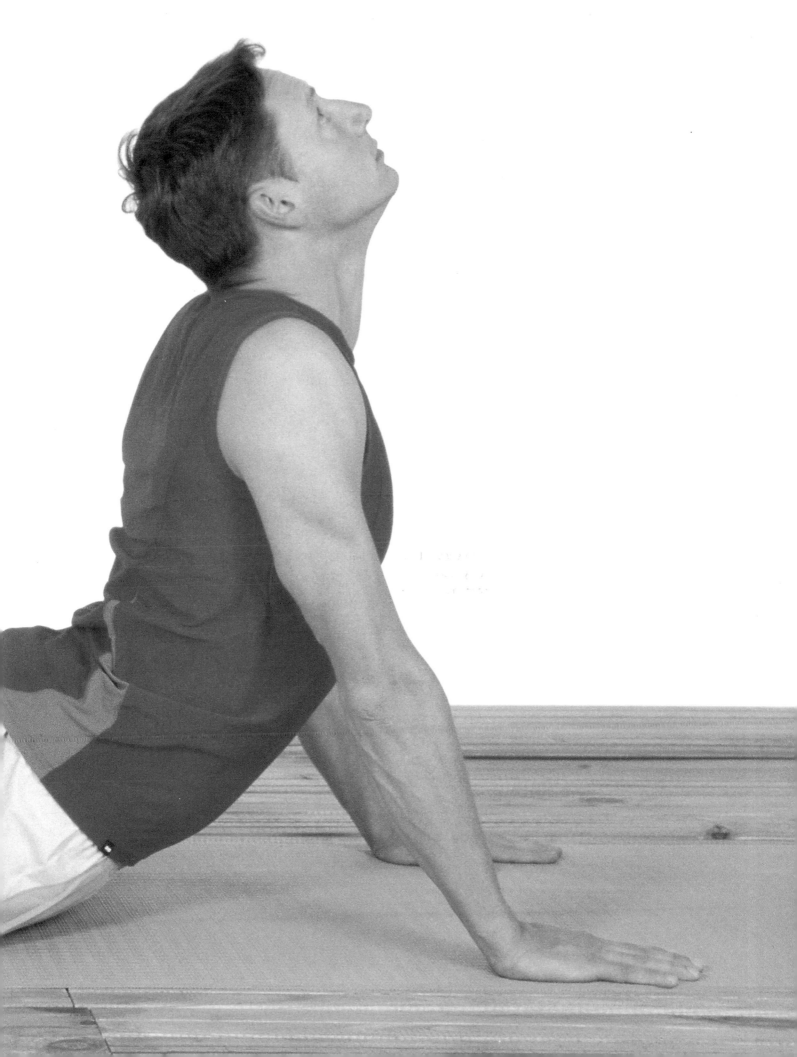

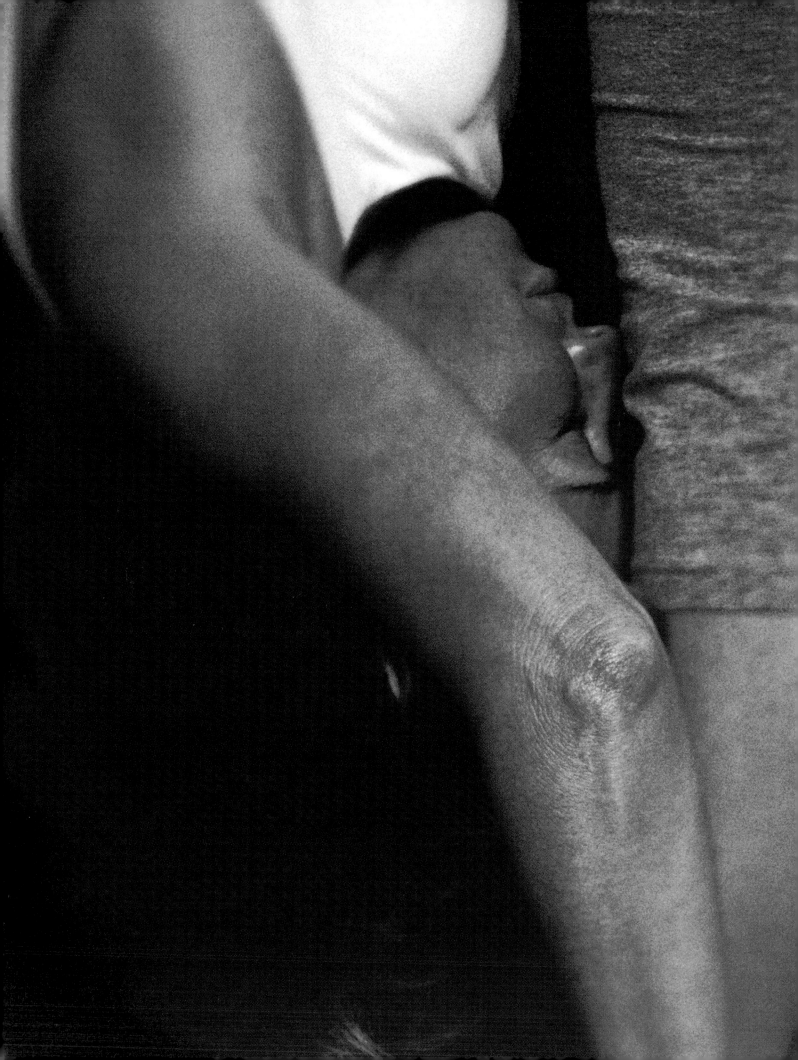

Contents

1

Introduction to Stretching

In the fast-moving world of today, three vital pieces of the health puzzle — relaxation, effective breathing and movement — are often overlooked, when spending as little as 10 minutes daily on these practices can improve overall health. There is no fast track to optimal relaxation, breathing and movement, but there is a way of combining them into one effective practice — that of flexibility training. More commonly known as stretching, it involves the movement of joints as well as the muscles that surround them. The method encouraged in this book allows for a deep level of relaxation, achieved through an effective breathing technique. Stretching can also be used to help alleviate stress, as a form of exercise, and for the improvement of posture and back health.

Stretching is one of the most important components of fitness — whether it is the only form of exercise you do, or whether you do it to supplement other forms of exercise, such as weight training, dancing, running or cycling, or to enhance performance in your chosen sport.

DEFINITIONS

Flexibility is a joint's ability to move freely through the full range of motion (ROM) allowed by its structure. This may involve movement in one plane only (hinge joints such as the knee), or movement in all directions (ball and socket joints such as the hip and shoulder). In order to achieve and maintain a joint's ROM, it is necessary to stretch the muscles that move those joints. **Static flexibility** is the ability to assume an extended position and then hold it still, whereas **dynamic flexibility** refers to the ability to use the muscles to move the joint through its range of motion.

- Helps achieve and maintain optimal joint ROM (range of movement) by lengthening the muscles, tendons (tissue that connects muscle to bone) and ligaments (tissue that connects bones) surrounding the joints.

- Helps improve posture, since it can aid in correcting muscle imbalances. For example, someone with excessively tight chest muscles may be pulled into a rounded back. This tends to stretch the back muscles out of their normal functional length. By stretching and thus loosening the tight muscles, the chest becomes more open and the back more upright.

- Helps correct muscle imbalance resulting from either poor posture or specific activities, which would pose an injury risk during even the mildest of physical activities.

- Can help reduce lower back (lumbar) pain. Stretches that target the muscles around the hips and pelvis may decrease the stress on the lumbar spine.

- Can help improve performance. For example, a hurdler needs flexible hips and a hiker needs flexible calf muscles and hamstrings.

- Aids mental and physical relaxation. Some forms of stretching promote deep, even and effective breathing, which can help clear the mind of negative, stressful thoughts. On the physiological level, an improved blood supply to the muscle reduces the accumulation of toxins – and thus fatigue. Also, longer (and thus looser) muscles are more relaxed than shorter (and tighter) muscles, hence flexibility promotes physical relaxation.

- Reduces muscle soreness resulting from exercise. Effective post-workout stretching relieves the muscles just used, and increases the blood and nutrient flow to them, thereby reducing the possibility, or severity, of delayed onset muscle soreness (DOMS).

- Stretching decreases the possibility of exceeding the extensibility (elasticity) of soft tissue during activity and thus injuring them.

- Indirectly helps to reduce susceptibility to muscle strain. Tight muscles can cause an imbalance in the body's alignment, which can result in muscle strain.

- Stretching increases blood and nutrient supply to the joint structures, muscles, tendons and ligaments, which may contribute to improved function and elasticity.

- Dynamic flexibility training (*see p23*) can reduce the time it takes for an impulse to travel to and from the brain, which improves neuromuscular coordination.

- Stretching can decrease muscle and joint fluid viscosity (thickness), resulting in smoother muscle contractions, and greater freedom of movement in the joint.

LIABILITIES OF INADEQUATE ROM

- increased risk of injury
- reduced functional capacity, for example, being unable to bend down or turn properly
- increased tension and reduced ability to relax

RIGHT: Flexibility training can be done anywhere, at any time – as long as your body is warm enough.

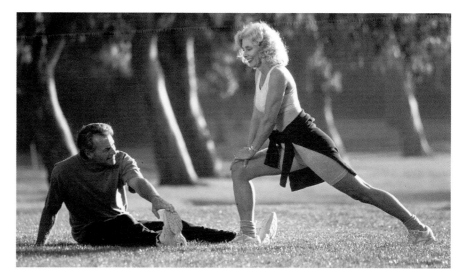

- premature ageing
- reduced performance in sports
- reduced muscle balance
- inability to optimize muscle contraction

FACTORS THAT AFFECT FLEXIBILITY

Joint structure

The joint structure determines the degree of free movement. Hinge joints, such as the knee or elbow, allow only flexion and extension (bending and straightening). Plane or gliding joints in the foot and hand consist of two flat surfaces that slide over each other. The saddle joint of the thumb allows two planes of motion. Pivot joints, such as the one at the base of the skull, facilitate rotational movement. Ball-and-socket joints, such as the hips and shoulders, allow the biggest range of movement.

Age

There appears to be a relationship between age and degree of flexibility, which tends to decrease gradually from the age of 25. Part of the ageing process is a certain amount of dehydration occurring in and around soft tissue, reducing lubrication and delivery of nutrients. However, flexibility can be developed at any age, and its decrease can be minimized by remaining active.

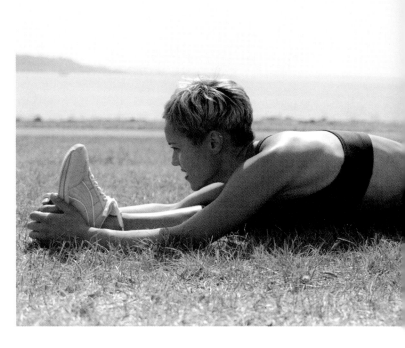

Gender

Although a generalization, females tend to be more flexible than males, possibly by genetic design to allow for increased flexibility in the pelvic region required during childbirth, for example.

Muscle mass

Many people believe that resistance training (leading to an increase in muscle mass) causes inflexibility, but this is not necessarily the case. Any physical activity programme, whether resistance training or even cardiovascular exercise, that does not include post-workout stretching, will result in a tight, inflexible body. However, a person who performs both resistance and flexibility training can become very supple.

Inactivity

Inactivity generally promotes adaptive shortening of the connective tissue. This leads to muscular imbalances, which is manifested in various ways, for example stooped shoulders, a hunched back (kyphosis) or an immobile spine. As a result even basic movements will cause discomfort, which in turn will also limit range of motion.

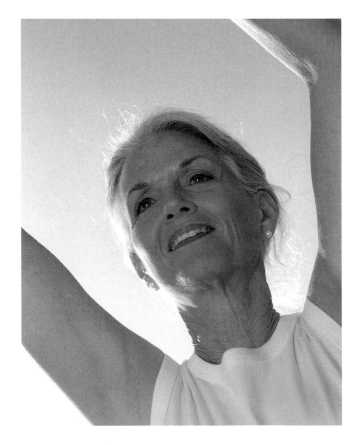

Flexibility can be developed at any age, minimizing the loss of mobility that goes with ageing.

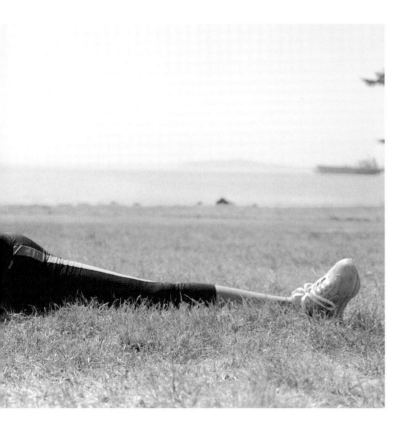

Some individuals are naturally more flexible than others, but a person's chosen activity will also determine the degree of flexibility that can be achieved.

Body type

There appears to be no scientific correlation between body type and degree of flexibility. More significant determinants are genetic make-up and a person's chosen activity. For instance, a typical ectomorph (a person with long, lean muscles) may achieve an extremely high degree of flexibility as a ballet dancer, but less so if the same person were a long distance runner

THE BROADER PICTURE

Fitness

Flexibility is one of the three main components of fitness, the other two being strength and cardiovascular fitness. While the latter is important for heart and lung health, strength and flexibility are vital for posture and physical efficiency.

A person engaged solely in strength work, at the expense of the other two components, would soon develop a body that is neither particularly fit nor functional because the muscles, although strong, would not allow movement through a full range of motion.

Concentrating only on flexibility training may result in a body that is unstable, due to an imbalance in strength versus flexibility.

Optimal fitness will not be achieved by someone neglecting cardio-vascular fitness.

A physical activity programme should ensure a balance between the three main components in order to contribute to wellness.

Wellness

Overall wellness requires not only a balanced physical activity programme, but also good nutrition, physical health and emotional wellbeing. In this context flexibility training contributes to wellness by requiring a person to be focused and controlled; to use slow, regular breathing; and to overcome the tendency to stay within one's comfort zone. It creates an opportunity for self-awareness and self-discovery.

Your body

Visualizing the targeted muscle gives focus to an exercise and helps concentration. Knowing what each muscle does can help you understand why you need to stretch it. For instance, tight muscles that cross a joint may be responsible for limiting the movement of that joint, and stretching them will diminish the tightness.

This section gives a brief summary of the name, location and function of most muscles, as well as the relevant joint/s crossed (if any).

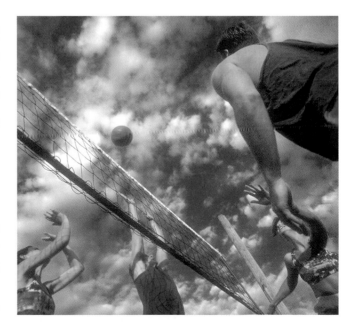

Balanced activity helps to lubricate the joints and thus contributes to maintaining range of motion.

THE FRONT VIEW SHOWING THE MAIN MUSCLES OF THE BODY

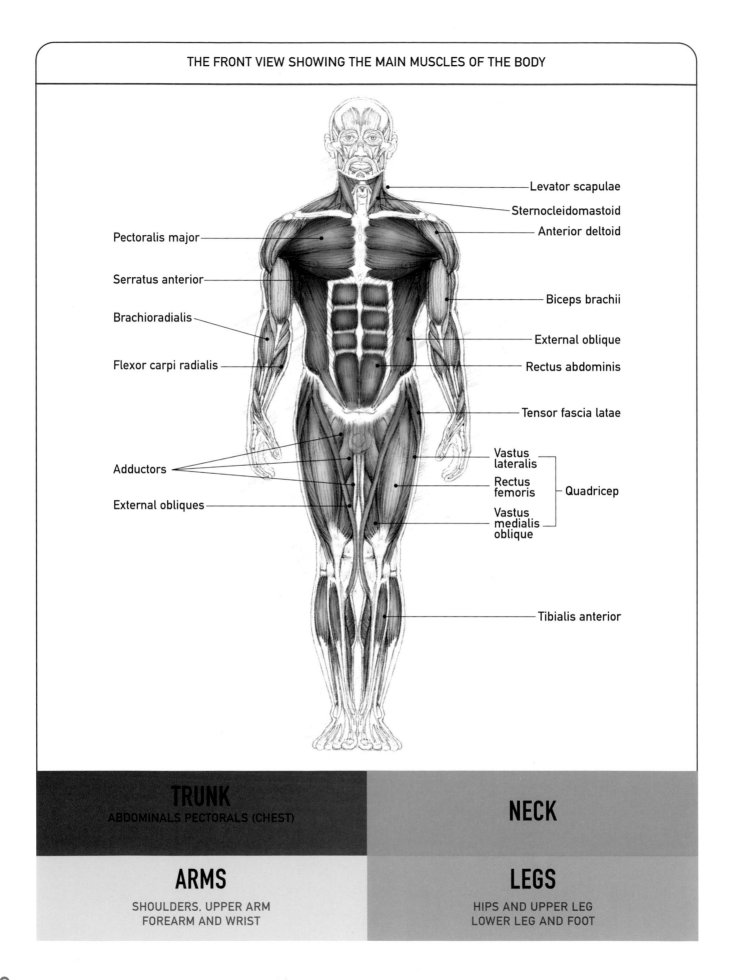

Pectoralis major

Serratus anterior

Brachioradialis

Flexor carpi radialis

Adductors

External obliques

Levator scapulae

Sternocleidomastoid

Anterior deltoid

Biceps brachii

External oblique

Rectus abdominis

Tensor fascia latae

Vastus lateralis

Rectus femoris

Vastus medialis oblique

Quadricep

Tibialis anterior

TRUNK
ABDOMINALS PECTORALS (CHEST)

NECK

ARMS

SHOULDERS, UPPER ARM
FOREARM AND WRIST

LEGS

HIPS AND UPPER LEG
LOWER LEG AND FOOT

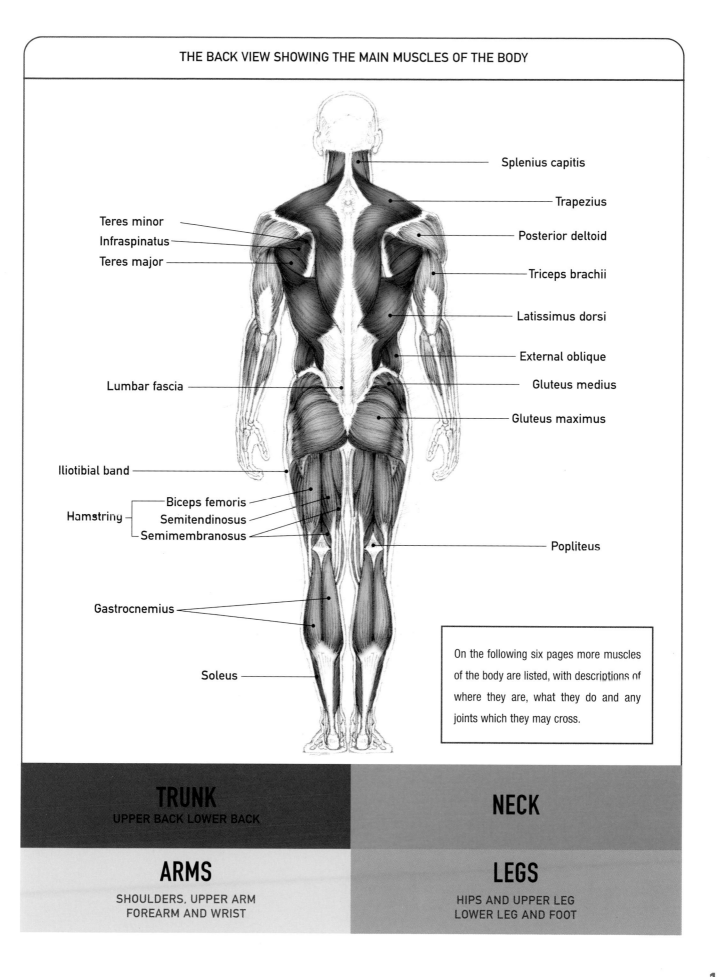

THE BACK VIEW SHOWING THE MAIN MUSCLES OF THE BODY

Splenius capitis

Trapezius

Teres minor

Infraspinatus

Teres major

Posterior deltoid

Triceps brachii

Latissimus dorsi

External oblique

Lumbar fascia

Gluteus medius

Gluteus maximus

Iliotibial band

Biceps femoris

Semitendinosus

Hamstring

Semimembranosus

Popliteus

Gastrocnemius

Soleus

On the following six pages more muscles of the body are listed, with descriptions of where they are, what they do and any joints which they may cross.

TRUNK
UPPER BACK LOWER BACK

NECK

ARMS
SHOULDERS, UPPER ARM
FOREARM AND WRIST

LEGS
HIPS AND UPPER LEG
LOWER LEG AND FOOT

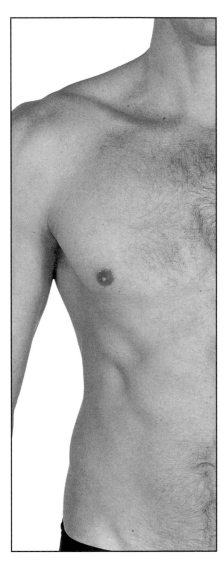

and bends the lower spine forward
Joint/s crossed: n/a

Pectoralis major

Location: in front of the first six ribs, as well as the sternum (breastbone) and the clavicle (collarbone)

Action: internally rotates the arms (movement is directed toward the front of the body within the transverse plane), moves them to the front of the body from a neutral position and draws them toward the body

Joint/s crossed: shoulder

Pectoralis minor

Location: front of the third, fourth and fifth ribs

Action: draws the shoulder blades away from one another and also assists in pushing them downward

Joint/s crossed: n/a

Serratus anterior

Location: surface of the ribs

Action: pulls the shoulder blades away from the spine

Joint/s crossed: n/a

1. Trunk (Front)

ABDOMINALS

Transverse abdominis

Location: deep into the abdominal region

Action: stabilizes the pelvis

Joint/s crossed: n/a

Internal and external obliques

Location: waist

Action: rotate the lower spine and bend it sideways and forward

Joint/s crossed: n/a

Rectus Abdominis

Location: front of ribs and pelvis

Action: flexes (bends) the spine to the side

2. Trunk (Back)

UPPER BACK

Trapezius

Location: upper, middle and lower back, close to the spine

Action: lifts, pushes down and pulls the shoulder blades together

Joint/s crossed: n/a

Rhomboid

Location: between shoulder blades

Action: pulls the shoulder blades together

Joint/s crossed: n/a

Teres major

Location: back of the lower portion of the shoulder blade

Action: lifts the arms backward, internally rotates them (movement is directed toward the front of the body within the transverse plane) and draws them toward the body

Joint/s crossed: shoulder

Teres minor

Location: back of the shoulder joint

Action: externally rotates the arm, moves it horizontally, away from the chest and lifts it backward

Joint/s crossed: shoulder

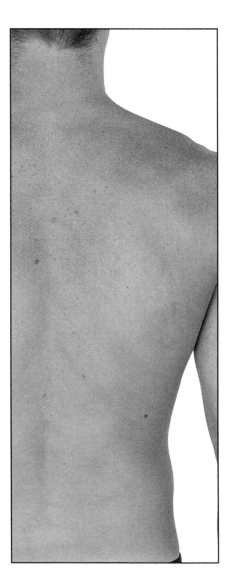

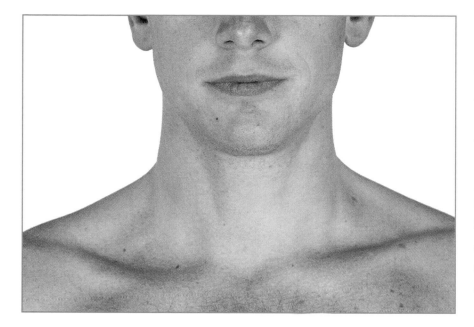

Erector spinae

Location: long muscles along the length of the spine

Action: extends the spine and bends it sideways

Joint/s crossed: n/a

3. Neck

Levator scapulae

Location: neck

Action: lifts the inside, top borders of the shoulder blades

Joint/s crossed: n/a

Splenius

Location: back of the neck

Action: tips the head and neck backward and rotates and bends both sideways

Joint/s crossed: n/a

Supraspinatus

Location: back of the top of the shoulder blade and humerus (upper arm bone)

Action: assists in lifting the arm sideways and stabilizes the head of the humerus in the glenoid cavity (which helps to stabilize this ball-and-socket joint)

Joint/s crossed: shoulder

Infraspinatus

Location: back of the middle of the shoulder blade

Action: externally rotates the arm, moves it horizontally away from the chest and lifts it backward

Joint/s crossed: shoulder

Subscapularis

Location: covers the underside of the shoulder blade

Action: internally rotates the arm, draws it downward toward the body and assists in lifting it backward

Joint/s crossed: shoulder

LOWER BACK

Quadratus lumborum

Location: lower back

Action: flexes the spine to the side and stabilizes the pelvis and lower (lumbar) spine

Joint/s crossed: n/a

Latissimus dorsi

Location: lower and middle back

Action: draws the arms toward the body, internally rotates them and moves them from the front of the body to the back

Joint/s crossed: shoulder

Sternocleidomastoid

Location: side of the base of the skull to front of collarbone and sternum

Action: tips the head forward and rotates and bends it sideways

Joint/s crossed: n/a

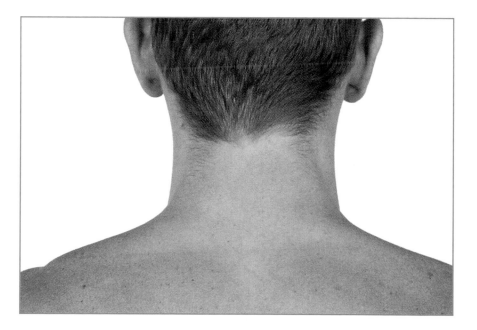

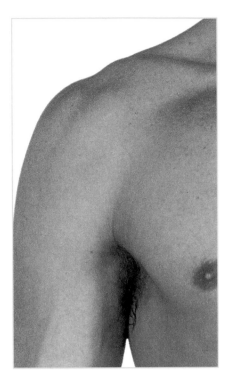

4. Arms

SHOULDERS

Deltoid

Location: shoulder

Action: lifts the arm sideways, forward and backward away from the body and rotates it both internally and externally

Joint/s crossed: shoulder

UPPER ARM

Triceps brachii

Location: back of the upper arm

Action: extends the elbow and lifts the arm backward away from the body

Joint/s crossed: shoulder and elbow

Biceps brachii

Location: front of the upper arm

Action: flexes the elbow, internally rotates the forearm and assists in moving the arm upward toward the front of the body

Joint/s crossed: shoulder and elbow

Coracobrachialis

Location: front of the shoulder

Action: lifts the arm forward, assists in drawing it toward the body and moves it horizontally across the chest

Joint/s crossed: shoulder

Brachioradialis

Location: forearm

Action: flexes the elbow and internally and externally rotates the forearm

Joint/s crossed: elbow

Brachialis

Location: lower half of the humerus

Action: flexes the elbow

Joint/s crossed: elbow

Anconeus

Location: inside the elbow joint

Action: extends the elbow joint

Joint/s crossed: elbow

Supinator

Location: outside the top of the forearm

Action: turns the hand and forearm so that the palm faces up or forward

Joint/s crossed: elbow

Pronator teres

Location: over the inside of the elbow joint

Action: internally rotates the forearm and assists in flexing the elbow

Joint/s crossed: elbow

Pronator quadratus

Location: inside of the wrist

Action: internally rotates the forearm

Joint/s crossed: n/a

FOREARM AND WRIST

In this section 'ulnar side of elbow joint' refers to the part of the elbow joint you would lean on if resting your arms on a table, the part where the ulnar interacts with the humerus (same side as that of your little finger). 'Radial side of elbow joint' refers to the opposite side, the part where the radius interacts with the humerus (same side as your thumb)

Flexor carpi radialis

Location: ulnar side of elbow joint to the point where first finger and thumb meet on the palm

Action: flexes the wrist (palm toward inside of forearm), pulls it sideways (thumb toward elbow joint) and assists with flexing the elbow

Joint/s crossed: elbow and wrist

Palmaris longus

Location: ulnar side of elbow joint to palm of the hand

Action: flexes the wrist (palm toward inside of forearm)

Joint/s crossed: elbow and wrist

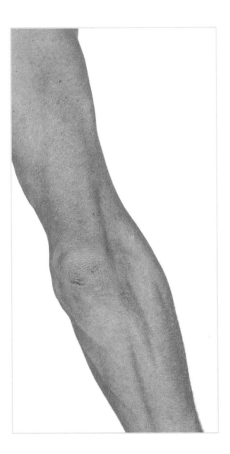

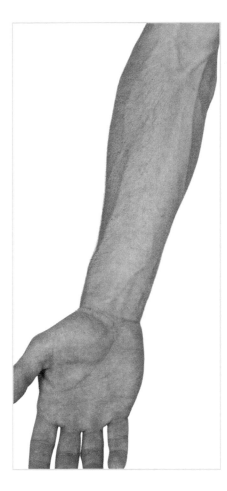

Flexor carpi ulnaris

Location: ulnar side of elbow joint to little finger-side of palm

Action: flexes the wrist (palm toward inside of forearm), pulls it sideways (little finger toward elbow joint) and assists with flexing the elbow

Joint/s crossed: elbow and wrist

Extensor carpi ulnaris

Location: radial side of elbow joint to baby finger side of back of hand

Action: extends the wrist (back of hand toward forearm), pulls it sideways (thumb toward elbow joint) and assists with extending the elbow

Joint/s crossed: elbow and wrist

Extensor carpi radialis brevis

Location: radial side of elbow joint to above middle finger on back of hand

Action: extends the wrist (back of hand toward forearm), pulls it sideways (little finger toward elbow joint) and assists with extending the elbow

Joint/s crossed: elbow and wrist

Extensor carpi radialis longus

Location: radial side of elbow joint to above second finger on back of the hand

Action: as above

Joint/s crossed: elbow and wrist

Flexor digitorum superficialis

Location: inside of forearm to fingers on the inside of the hand

Action: flexes the fingers and wrist (palm toward forearm), and assists with flexing the elbow

Joint/s crossed: elbow and wrist

Flexor digitorum profundus

Location: inside of forearm to fingers on the inside of the hand

Action: same as above, but without flexing of the elbow

Joint/s crossed: elbow and wrist

Flexor pollicis longus

Location: thumb side of forearm to the end of the thumb

Action: flexes thumb and wrist (palm toward forearm)

Joint/s crossed: wrist

Extensor digitorum

Location: radial side of elbow joint to fingers on back of hand

Action: extends the wrist and fingers (back of the hand and fingers toward the forearm) and assists with extending the elbow

Joint/s crossed: elbow and wrist

Extensor indicis

Location: halfway down outside of forearm to end of first finger

Action: extends the first finger (back of the finger toward the forearm) and assists with extending the wrist (back of the hand toward the forearm)

Joint/s crossed: wrist

Extensor digiti minimi

Location: radial side of elbow joint to end of little finger

Action: extends the little finger (back of the finger toward the forearm) and assists with extending the wrist (back of the hand toward the forearm)

Joint/s crossed: elbow and wrist

Extensor pollicis longus

Location: halfway down the outside of the forearm to the end of the thumb

Action: extends the thumb and wrist (back of thumb and hand toward the outside of the forearm)

Joint/s crossed: wrist

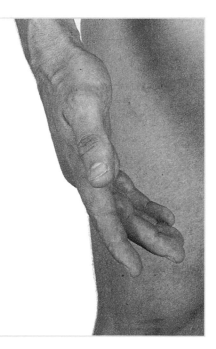

Extensor pollicis brevis

Location: halfway down the outside of the forearm to halfway down the thumb

Action: as above

Joint/s crossed: wrist

Abductor pollicis longus

Location: halfway down the outside of the forearm to the base of the thumb

Action: pulls the wrist and the thumb sideways (thumb and hand toward the elbow joint)

Joint/s crossed: wrist

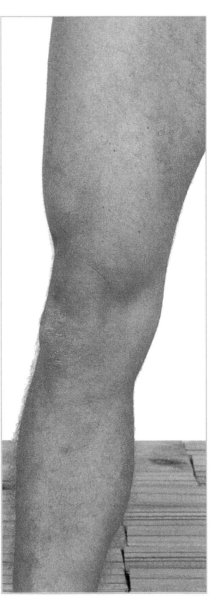

5. Legs

HIPS AND UPPER LEG

Iliopsoas

Location: front of pelvis

Action: flexes the hip and externally rotates the leg (the movement is toward the back of the body)

Joint/s crossed: hip

Sartorius

Location: starts at the outside of the hip and ends just beyond the inside of the knee

Action: flexes the hip and the knee and externally rotates the leg at the same time

Joint/s crossed: hip and knee

Quadriceps

Location: front of thigh

Action: flexes the hip and extends the knee

Joint/s crossed: hip and knee

Tensor fasciae latae

Location: outside of the leg

Action: pulls the leg away from the body, flexes the hip and rotates the leg internally at the same time

Joint/s crossed: hip and knee

Gluteus medius

Location: side of buttocks

Action: pulls the leg away from the body and both externally and internally rotates it

Joint/s crossed: hip

Gluteus maximus

Location: buttocks

Action: extends the hip and externally rotates the legs

Joint/s crossed: hip

Gluteus minimus

Location: side of buttocks

Action: pulls the leg away from the body

Joint/s crossed: hip

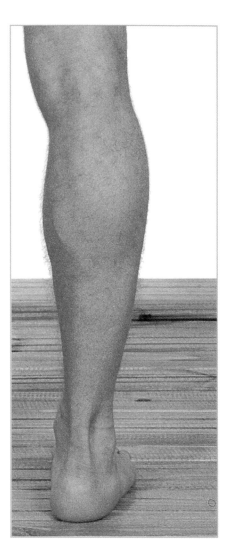

Rotator group (piriformis, gemellus superior and inferior, obturator externus and internus, quadratus femoris)

Location: buttocks

Action: external rotation of the hip (leg)

Joint/s crossed: hip

Hamstring

Location: back of leg

Action: flexes the knee, externally and internally rotates the leg and extends the hip

Joint/s crossed: hip and knee

Pectineus

Location: front of the pubis

Action: flexes the hip, internally rotates the

leg and draws the leg toward the body
Joint/s crossed: hip

Adductors
Location: inner thigh
Action: draws the leg toward the body, externally rotates it and assists in flexing the hip
Joint/s crossed: hip

Gracilis
Location: inner thigh
Action: draws the leg toward the body, flexes the knee and internally rotates the leg (movement directed toward front of the body)
Joint/s crossed: hip and knee

Popliteus
Location: behind the knee
Action: flexes and internally rotates the knee
Joint/s crossed: knee

LOWER LEG AND FOOT

Gastrocnemius
Location: calf
Action: extends (points) the ankle and flexes the knee
Joint/s crossed: knee and ankle

Soleus
Location: calf
Action: extends the ankle
Joint/s crossed: knee and ankle

Tibialis anterior
Location: from the shin into the foot
Action: flexes the ankle (pulls the toes toward the shin) and rolls the foot outward
Joint/s crossed: ankle

Tibialis posterior
Location: From the calf into the foot

Action: extends ankle and rolls foot outward
Joint/s crossed: ankle

Flexor digitorum longus
Location: from the calf into the foot
Action: extends the ankle, rolls the top of the foot outward and extends the four lesser toes
Joint/s crossed: ankle

Flexor hallucis longus
Location: from the calf into the foot
Action: extends the ankle, rolls the top of the foot outward and extends the big toe
Joint/s crossed: ankle

Peroneus longus
Location: from the outside of the calf into the foot
Action: extends the ankle and rolls the top of the foot inward
Joint/s crossed: ankle

Peroneus brevis
Location: from the outside of the lower calf into the foot
Action: extends the ankle and rolls the top of the foot inward
Joint/s crossed: ankle

Peroneus tertius
Location: from the outside of the ankle into the foot
Action: flexes the ankle and rolls the top of the foot inward
Joint/s crossed: ankle

Extensor digitorum longus
Location: from the outside of shin into the foot
Action: flexes the ankle, rolls the foot inward and extends the four lesser toes
Joint/s crossed: ankle

Extensor hallucis longus
Location: from the outside of the shin into the foot
Action: flexes the ankle, assists in rolling the foot inward and extends the big toe
Joint/s crossed: ankle

External rotation: The outward rotation of a joint. The movement is directed toward the back of the body.

Internal rotation: The inward rotation of a joint. Movement is directed toward the front of the body.

Movement in the Transverse plane: Movement in the horizontal direction (parallel to the ground)

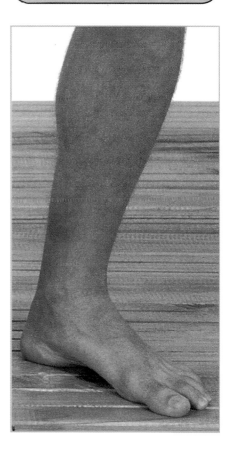

GOOD TO KNOW

Apparel

No doubt you'll wear the clothes in which you feel most comfortable, but you also need to consider moisture absorption, climate and shape when choosing your workout attire.

Start with stretch. Choose a fabric that moves with your body (imagine trying to perform the splits in a pair of jeans). Most gym wear is made to allow for that, with an emphasis on comfort (and, like it or not, fashion).

Cotton, being a natural fibre, absorbs sweat well and is comfortable against the skin. If you do not sweat a great deal, stretch cotton apparel will be fine. If you do sweat a lot, this fibre tends to hold moisture and does not dry quickly, which means that you may be working out in soggy clothing. In that case, a nylon/spandex fibre, which dries really quickly, will be better. There are also 'moisture management' fabrics that have been treated with a finish, causing the clothing to act as though it were a natural fabric in terms of sweat absorption. The same effect is also offered by fabrics that have been specially constructed, as opposed to treated.

Another option available to you is a new generation synthetic called Microfibre (also in combination with spandex). Apart from feeling far more luxurious against the skin, it has enhanced moisture management properties.

Anti-bacterial fabrics are useful in situations where, for example, you are unable to shower immediately after your workout.

The second consideration when choosing workout apparel is climate. While it is more effective stretching in warmer rather then cooler temperatures, you don't want to make yourself hotter than you need to be, so wear short-sleeved, short-legged clothing which is light and porous. Equally, if the weather's cool, you'll definitely want to maintain body heat, so long-sleeved, long-legged clothing made of thicker fabric would be best. A beanie or woolly hat wouldn't go amiss either.

The third consideration is shape. Whether you're choosing to join a group stretch class, attend a private session with an instructor, or simply work in front of your mirror at home, it can help (either the teacher or yourself) tremendously to see what's happening to the line of your body while you stretch. Although this doesn't mean you need to be kitted out in the latest breathtakingly tight stretch gear, you should give some thought to wearing non-baggy clothing.

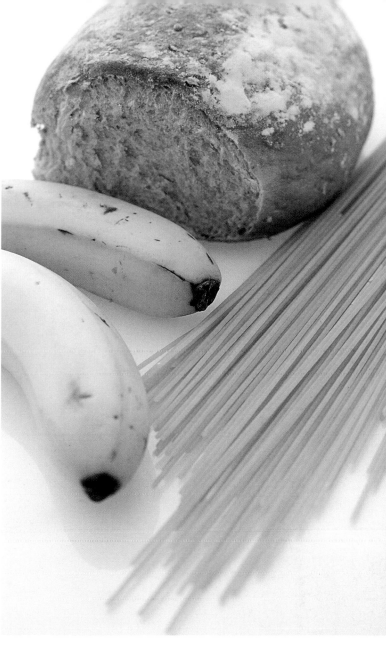

Hydration

Water intake during flexibility training sessions is a very subjective issue. If you tend to sweat a great deal during your workouts, you will want to keep a water bottle with you and try to drink at regular intervals throughout the session. Even if you do not sweat a great deal but feel comfortable drinking during this type of workout, or if it's a really hot day, it is recommended that you do the same.

A good way to establish whether or not you are dehydrated is by the colour of your urine. A hydrated body shows pale yellow or clear urine, while a dehydrated one shows dark yellow urine. Tea, coffee and alcohol are all diuretics and thus dehydrate the body, even though your urine may look clear, so if you drink a lot of these beverages make sure you drink additional water. In general, six to eight glasses daily of good quality water should be fine, unless you are particularly active (in which case, more should be taken). Water is usually adequate, but if you will be taking part in an intense stretch session for longer than an hour, you may consider some form of sports drink, which supplies energy and electrolytes and encourages further fluid intake.

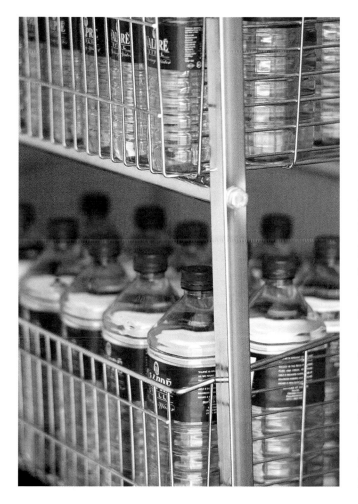

Food

How soon before or after exercise you should eat depends on personal preference and the intensity of the workout. It is best not to eat anything substantial for at least two hours before high intensity physical activity (such as a really stringent yoga class), or anything that requires lots of abdominal work, or bending at the waist.

Carbohydrates are used to replenish fuel used up during your workout and their absorption appears to be most efficient shortly after exercise. Protein is put to use repairing and building muscle (among other things) after exercise. For that reason it is best to eat something containing protein and carbohydrates within two hours after a high intensity workout.

If, of course, your workout wasn't particularly taxing, go with what feels comfortable for you or wait for hunger signals (often exercise can block hunger pangs for a while after you have completed a session).

The Science of Stretching

2

In order to fully understand why one should participate in a programme of flexibility training, it would help to have knowledge of the physiology involved in the action of stretching your body. In this way, you can apply the science of stretching to the practice of lengthening your muscles both efficiently and effectively.

In this chapter you will also learn how to assess your own body through a series of postural tests, the results of which can be used to design your own personalized stretching programme.

THE STRETCH REFLEX

The stretch reflex is the muscle's response to a sudden, unexpected increase in its length. Muscles contain proprioceptors – nerve endings that detect changes in physical displacement and changes in tension or force within the body. When a muscle is stretched rapidly, one of these, the muscle spindle, sends out an impulse that initiates a converse reflex action, namely, to contract the muscle. The more sudden the change in muscle length and, up to a point, the harder a muscle is stretched, the stronger the reflex contraction. The basic function of the muscle spindle is to help maintain muscle tone and prevent injury. For this reason the old practice of bouncing to increase a stretch is counter-productive and can lead to injury (*see also 'Ballistic' on opposite page*).

When tension exceeds a certain threshold, however, the golgi tendon organ sends a signal to stop the contraction, allowing the muscle to relax. The sudden relaxation is a protective mechanism to prevent tendons and muscles being torn away from their attachments. Careful, controlled static stretching makes use of this reflex to improve flexibility (*see under the heading 'Static' on the opposite page*).

METHODS OF STRETCHING

There are a number of techniques used for flexibility training. Some are used specifically by athletes to optimize their performance, while others are used in various medical disciplines to rehabilitate damaged muscles, tendons or ligaments. Yet other techniques are more appropriate for anyone simply wanting to achieve a state of postural and muscular balance.

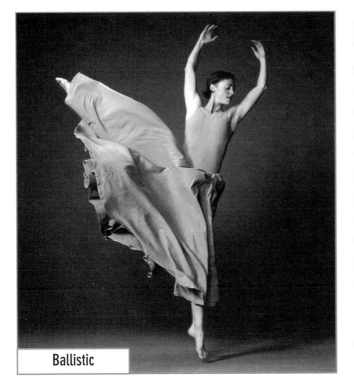

Ballistic

3. Static

This method involves a slow, gradual and controlled stretch, which is then held. This reduces the muscle's reflex action and instead facilitates the golgi tendon organ (*see 'Stretch Reflex' opposite page*), allowing the muscle to lengthen without risk of injury. Although an unfit, inflexible person may experience post-stretch muscle soreness with this method, it will ease with practice. When performing the numbered stretches in this book, it is recommended that you use the static stretching technique, since it is also excellent for relaxation. More advice will be given in Chapter 3 regarding exercise execution. There are other techniques that are grouped with static stretching, although most of them require a partner. Examples are: passive, active assistive and proprioceptive neuromuscular facilitation (PNF).

PASSIVE

This requires, as it sounds, a person to remain passive and relaxed, making no contribution to the range of motion, while a partner applies the necessary force to stretch the appropriate body part (*see below*).

ABOVE: Dance movements often require dancers to swing one leg as high as they can, while standing on the other. While it is a good example of ballistic stretching, it is not recommended for untrained individuals.

1. Ballistic

This method of stretching involves rapid, uncontrolled bouncing or jerking movements. It takes the muscle to its fullest range of movement and then adds momentum or weight to the motion (for example dancers swinging one leg as high as they can while standing on the other). However, there is the risk of loading soft tissue structures beyond their normal capabilities, leading to injury. Also, the muscle spindle may be activated, causing a reflex contraction, which can put the muscle at further risk of tearing and also putting ligaments and tendons at risk. Although used by trained individuals such as dancers, it is not recommended for use by the general population.

2. Dynamic

Although sometimes confused with ballistic stretching, this technique can also be described as mobilization stretching. Dynamic stretching consists of controlled movement that takes you gently to the limits of your range of motion, whereas ballistic stretches involve trying to force a part of the body beyond its range of motion. In dynamic stretches there are no bounces or jerky movements,

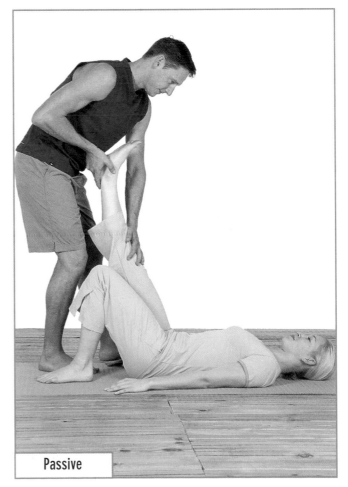

Passive

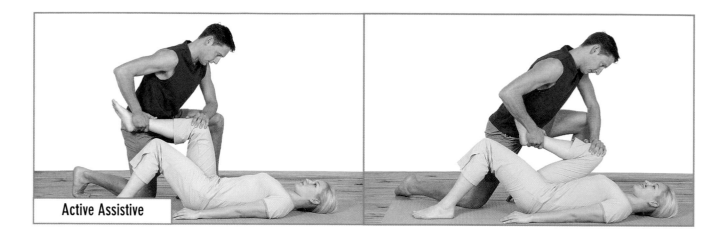

Active Assistive

ACTIVE ASSISTIVE

This technique also requires a partner, and is used when, due to weakness, the muscle or joint being stretched may need assistance through its range of movement.

PROPRIOCEPTIVE NEUROMUSCULAR FACILITATION (PNF)

Originally developed for use in physiotherapy, PNF can lead to considerable improvements in flexibility. A partner is required to assist the person stretching. The relevant muscle (for instance, the back of the leg) is taken to its fullest range (perhaps 90° off the floor while you're lying on your back), followed by a six- to 10-second contraction of the same muscle against a resistance, while still in the stretch (the partner pushing your leg further toward your head while you push back). This is followed by relaxation in the same range. This process is repeated two or three times.

The benefit of this technique is that it stimulates the golgi tendon organ's response to allow further stretching of the muscle. It is frequently used around ball and socket joints, such as the hips and shoulders.

WHEN NOT TO STRETCH

The American College of Sports Medicine (ACSM) advises against stretching an area when there is:

- a bone blocking motion
- an unhealed fracture
- infection and/or acute inflammation affecting the joint or surrounding tissue
- sharp pain associated with the stretch or uncontrolled muscle cramping when attempting to stretch
- local haematoma (bruising/swelling) as a result of an injury caused by overstretching
- the need for a shortened muscle to provide stability to a joint capsule or ligament
- intentional muscle contraction to improve function or to compensate for a disability (people with paralysis or severe muscle weakness may use, for example, the tightness in a finger muscle to pick up objects).

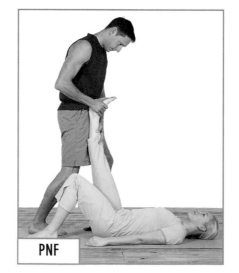

PNF

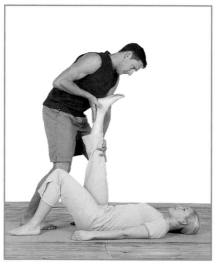

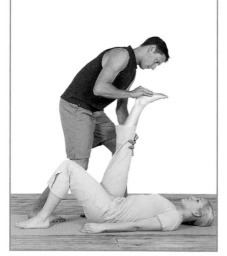

Some people are hypermobile, with naturally loose muscles, ligaments and tendons allowing excessive ROM. Since it is important to maintain joint stability, these individuals should not stretch into the extremes of this ROM.

During pregnancy, hormones are released which increase joint range of motion through laxness in the ligaments and muscles. For this reason excessive stretching is not recommended during this period.

LIABILITIES OF EXCESSIVE FLEXIBILITY

There is a trade-off between flexibility and stability. Excessive flexibility reduces the support offered to the joints by their adjacent muscles and increases the risk of injury. Also, once a muscle has been stretched to its maximum, attempting to increase the stretch will only stretch the ligaments and put undue stress on the tendons, neither of which should be stretched. (Tendons are not supposed to lengthen and ligaments will tear when stretched more than six per cent of their normal length.)

Instability may lead to a reduction in the reflexes that protect the joints and a decrease in neuromuscular coordination. This could also increase the risk of joint degenerative conditions, such as arthritis.

WHEN SHOULD I STRETCH?

Because our bodies tend to become more flexible with movement through the day, it makes sense to stretch in the evenings, or some time during the day. First thing in the morning one usually experiences some stiffness caused by fairly immobile sleep positions. However, it may be the only time you have for stretching. The most important thing is that you do take the time to stretch.

HOW SHOULD IT FEEL?

Some stretches may feel uncomfortable initially, but try to stay in them, even if only for a short while. As long as you feel no pain, you should not be in danger of injuring yourself. Don't bounce your stretch. Breathe

GOOD TO KNOW

Warming Up

Always warm up before stretching. This prepares the body for the activity ahead by slowly increasing your heart rate. This speeds up the blood supply, and oxygen from haemoglobin, to the working muscles. It also speeds up your metabolic rate and the speed at which nerve impulses travel (making movement easier). It increases tissue temperature and decreases muscle tightness or tension. This phase of a workout improves the muscle's ability to contract and relax, and the connective tissue's ability to elongate. It gives the body an opportunity to adapt comfortably to an increased workload.

An effective warm-up should leave you feeling warm, but not out of breath. On a cold day your warm-up may take as long as 10 minutes, whereas in warmer weather five minutes may suffice.

THERE ARE THREE WAYS TO WARM UP

1. A general warm-up involves any activity that requires regular movement of your largest muscle groups (legs, torso and buttocks). Some examples are cycling, walking, climbing stairs, even doing some light push-ups, lunges or squats.
2. A passive warm-up involves 'cheating' by increasing the body's temperature without physical activity, for example a warm bath or heat packs.
3. In some cases a routine is used that prepares the body more specifically by mimicking the movements to be done in the work-out. In yoga, for example, the sun salutation comprises a variety of specific stretches and poses that flow together, ensuring constant movement throughout the warm-up.

As with any physical activity programme, be sure to progress slowly. If at any stage you feel distress or pain, stop immediately and seek professional advice.

calmly, regularly and through your nose. Consciously try to relax your body, since the looser you are, the easier you will feel in the stretch and the deeper you'll be able to take it. Go to the point of mild discomfort, but not pain; try for a rating of 3–7 on a scale of 1–10.

HOW OFTEN AND HOW LONG?

Initially you may only be able to hold your stretches for a few seconds, but to increase muscle length and to initiate the relaxation response, a stretch should be held for between 30 and 90 seconds.

Your flexibility goals will determine how often you stretch. This could be twice a week or every day. If your aim is to counter postural tightness (for example, lower back pain or neck stiffness related to muscular inflexibility), then try to stretch every day.

Stretching can help alleviate the discomfort associated with long periods of immobility, for example, when travelling. In that case you might do a few gentle stretches at intervals throughout the day.

Stretching at intervals during the day – in the office, while watching television or reading a book – can be beneficial as long as it is done with awareness and good form.

WHAT TO LOOK OUT FOR

It is important to maintain good postural alignment while stretching. In order to help you understand optimal alignment for each of the stretches described in Chapter 3, and because it is quite possible (in fact, relatively easy) to injure yourself when stretching incorrectly, some cues for good technique will be given, with warnings on how not to perform the stretch.

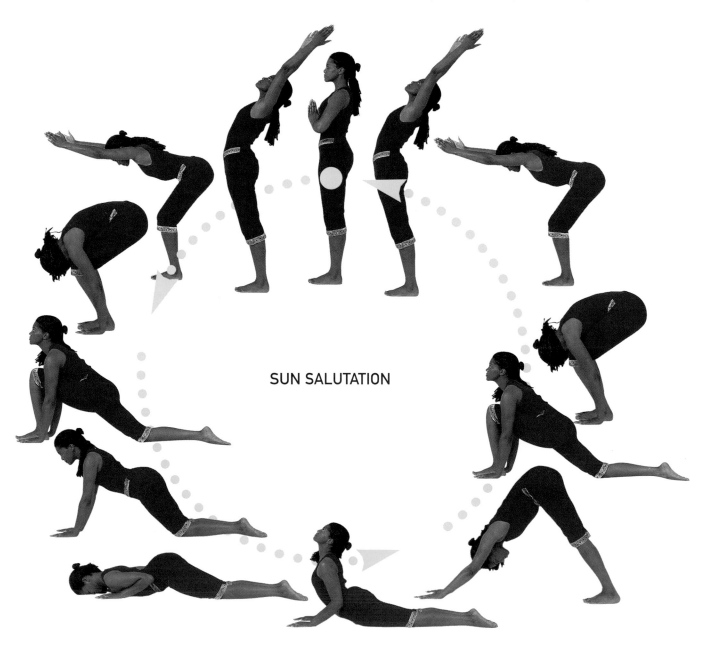

SUN SALUTATION

SELF-ASSESSMENT

The following assessment is a fairly basic one in that it will give you an indication of your general flexibility in the limbs and trunk. Keep in mind, however, that if you need to establish specific flexibility issues, you will need a professional assessment. This would include an evaluation of the strength in opposing muscle groups, because when muscles cause a limb to move through the joint's range of motion, they usually act in cooperating groups. An imbalance will have an effect on flexibility.

Use the outcome of this assessment together with the information in Chapter 1 (Your body) and Chapter 3 (The menu of stretches) to create your own unique stretch programme.

Trunk

TEST 1: PELVIS

Stand sideways in front of a mirror in what feels like a naturally relaxed position (don't change your posture if you think it is faulty). Place two fingers of the hand furthest from the mirror on your pubic bone (make sure you can actually feel the bone). Place two fingers of the other hand on top of the hip bone of the leg closest to the mirror.

If the fingers on your hip bone are in front of the fingers on your pubic bone, it indicates anterior pelvic tilt. If they are behind the pubic bone, it indicates posterior pelvic tilt. If your fingers are in line with each other it indicates a neutral posture.

If your pelvis is held in an anterior tilt, you would benefit from doing stretches for the lower back, since it is usually arched in people with this posture. You may also benefit from stretches of the hip flexor muscles (iliopsoas), which are often flexed in this case.

If your pelvis is held in a posterior tilt, you should include some stretches for the abdominals, which are normally contracted in this type of posture, and for the hamstrings, also often contracted.

With correct posture, the pelvis lies in a neutral position, neither forward nor back.

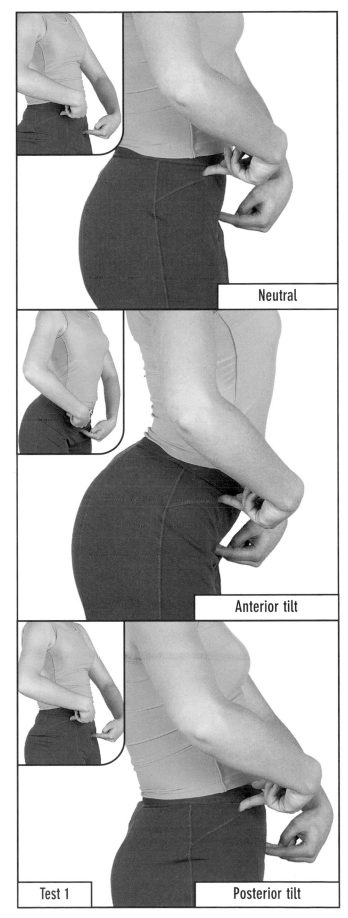

Neutral

Anterior tilt

Test 1

Posterior tilt

TEST 2: SPINE FLEXIBILITY/MOBILITY

Sit on a chair, placed sideways to a mirror, so that you can see the shape of your spine. With your knees bent, lean forward slowly and attempt to rest your chest on your thighs.

When you've reached the point where your trunk stops moving forward, look sideways in the mirror and take note of whether your upper, middle and lower spine is rounded or straight.

If your trunk touches your thighs in this forward-leaning position and is rounded in all three areas of the back, it indicates that you do not have a problem with tight back extensors nor with tight posterior leg muscles, which cross the hip joint and can affect lower back flexibility. This is good news, since lower back pain frequently stems from compression (caused by tightness) of the vertebral discs in this area of the spine.

If any particular area shows tightness and does not curve easily, this would be the area on which to concentrate in your flexibility programme.

To maintain good posture, you should stretch all the muscles that cross the hip joint, as well as those on the back of the trunk.

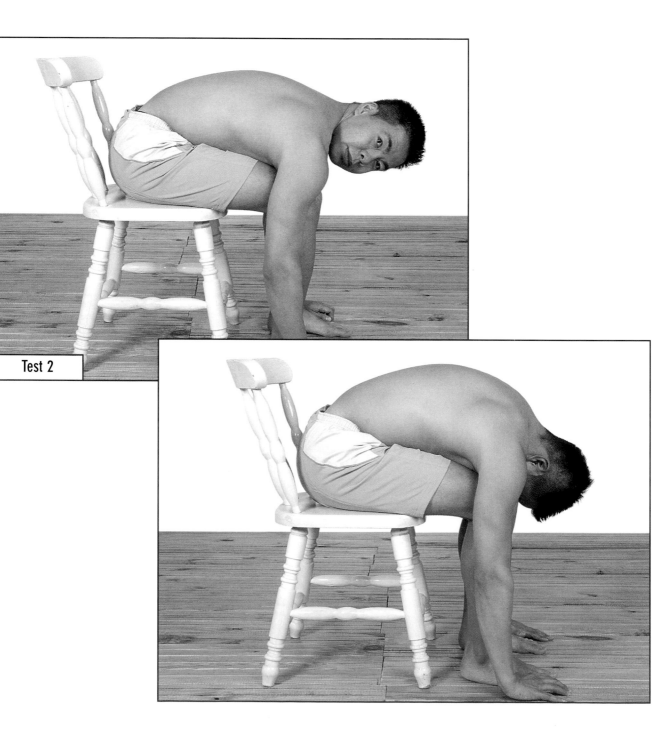

Test 2

TEST 3: SPINE FLEXIBILITY/MOBILITY

Sit on a stool, sideways to a mirror. Elongate your spine and extend it backward as much as possible without rolling the pelvis forward. Look in the mirror to see the shape of your spine.

Is your upper, middle and lower spine concave or straight?

If you can see stiffness in any area of the spine, you should select stretches for that particular area from those for the lower, middle and upper back in Chapter 3.

TEST 4: PECTORALS (CHEST)

Stand in a relaxed manner sideways to the mirror and look at the position of your shoulders in relation to your chest. Do your shoulders droop forward (roll inward) or is your chest open, with shoulders drawn lightly backward?

If your shoulders droop forward ✱, a possible reason is that your chest muscles are tight. Although there may also be other contributing factors, such as a weak serratus anterior muscle, it is recommended that you do the stretches given for the chest area.

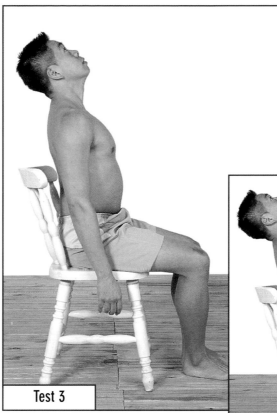

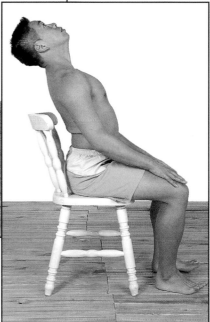

Test 3

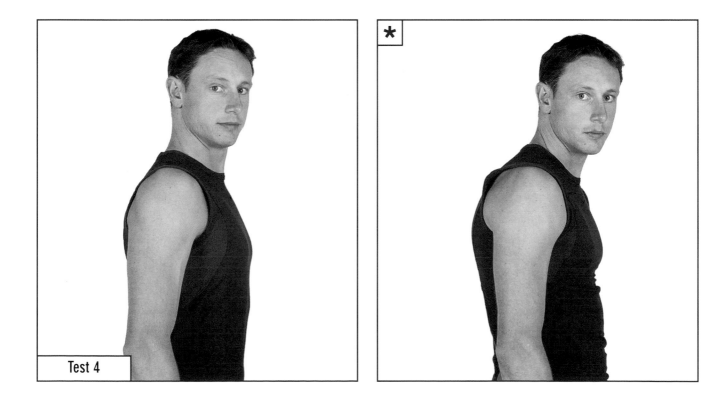

Test 4

✱

TEST 5: RHOMBOIDS (UPPER BACK)

Stand side on to the mirror, with a slight turn, so that you have a better view of your back and shoulder blades. Better still, ask a partner to stand behind you and look at your shoulders. Are your shoulder blades drawn together, or are they lying flat against your back? The optimal position of the shoulder blades is approximately 5½cm (2in) from the spine.

If they are retracted (drawn together), your rhomboid muscles may be tight, so include stretches for this area of the middle back.

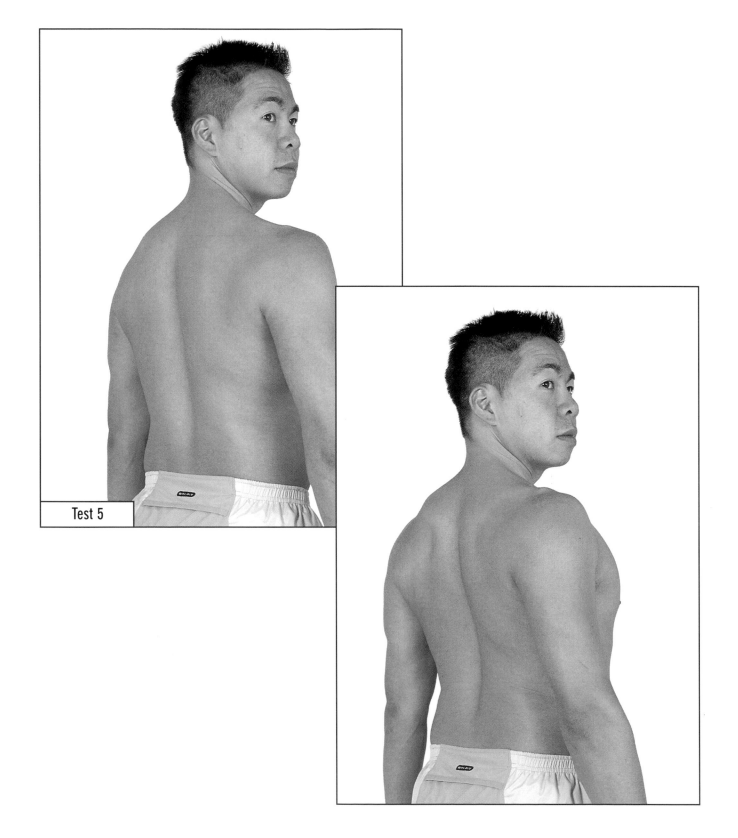

Test 5

TEST 6: MIDDLE AND UPPER BACK

Lie on the floor with your legs bent, feet on the floor, and arms at your side. Keeping your navel pulled in toward your spine, raise your arms above your chest with the palms facing your feet. Slowly lower the hands toward the floor behind your head, without arching your lower back.

If you are loose in the middle and upper back muscles, you will probably be flexible enough to be able to touch the floor with the backs of your hands. If you are unable to do so without arching your lower back ✶, then they may be somewhat tight and you should include stretches from the menu in Chapter 3 for this part of the back.

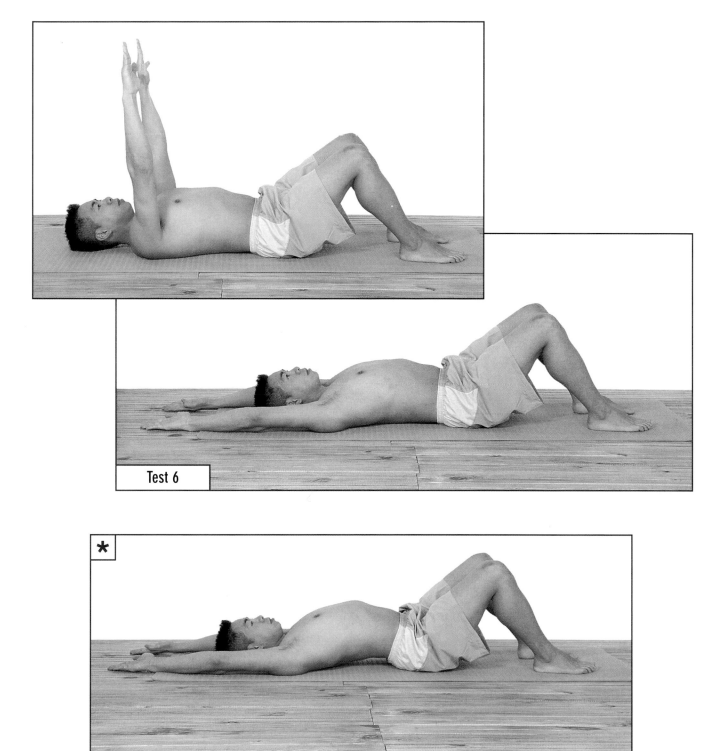

Test 6

✶

Neck

TEST 7: NECK 1

Sit or stand and drop your head forward. Your chin should touch your chest. If not, do some stretches for the back of the neck.

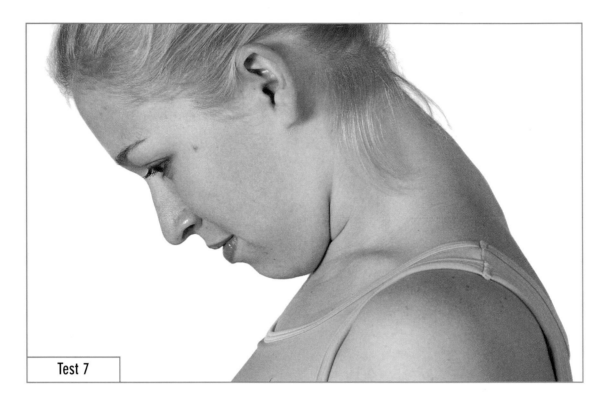

Test 7

TEST 8: NECK 2

Drop your head to the side and note how far you can go and how it feels.

Stiffness in this area will be quite uncomfortable, in which case you need to add some side neck stretches to your programme.

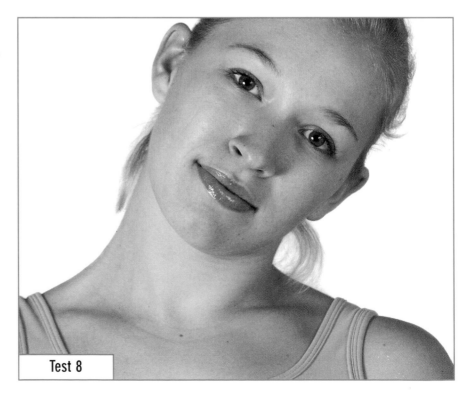

Test 8

Arms

TEST 9: SHOULDERS 1

Sit or stand and take your left arm behind your back, palm facing away from your back and elbow bent so that your fingers point up your spine. Stretch your right arm up to the ceiling, bend the elbow and bring the hand down, with the palm facing your back to clasp the right hand. Repeat on the other side.

If your hands touch on both sides your shoulder flexibility is good. If not, try to establish where you feel the tightness. It may be in the back of the raised arm, in which case you need to include stretches for the triceps. If the stiffness is in the front of the shoulder of the bottom arm (this can be very uncomfortable), then choose stretches for the deltoid muscle.

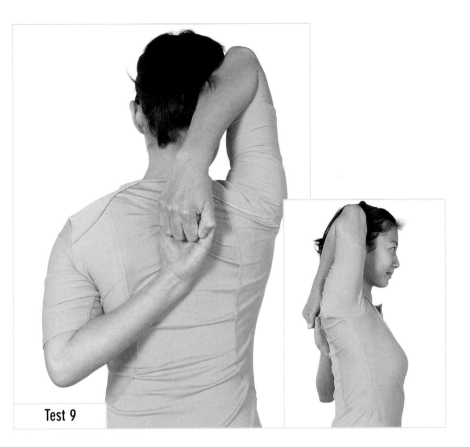

Test 9

TEST 10: SHOULDERS 2

Stand, take your arms up to the ceiling, keeping them close to the ears with your elbows straight, palms facing each other. Contract your abdominals and pull your ribs back toward your spine to avoid arching the lower back. Lower your arms and take them behind your back as far as possible without rolling your shoulders forward. When your arms are up, and they are not directly above your shoulders and in line with your ears, but angled forward slightly, you could have a combination of shoulder and back tightness, especially the latissimus dorsi. If, when taking your arms behind your body, you are unable to lift them without rolling your shoulders forward ⭐, and without the arms splaying to the side as they are raised, you may have a combination of shoulder and chest tightness. Either way, some shoulder stretches would be worth doing.

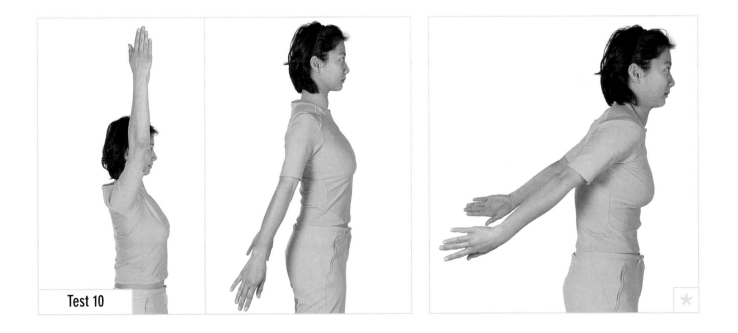

Test 10

Hips and Legs

TEST 11: HAMSTRINGS
(BACK OF LEGS)

Sit on the ground with your legs straight ahead of you, hands at your sides and toes pointing up to the ceiling. If you are unable to maintain an upright spine and pelvis (and instead roll back in the pelvis or round the lower back), you may have tight hamstrings.

Although it is possible that you may also be tight in the lower back, you would have established this with the first test, under the heading Trunk. If you felt any stiffness in your calves while in this position, you could add some calf stretches to your programme.

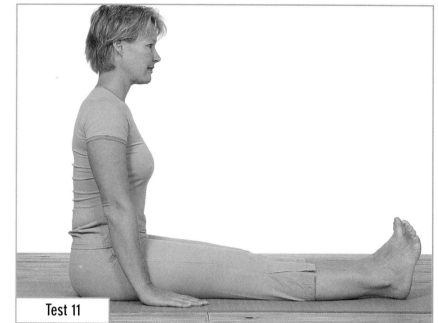

Test 11

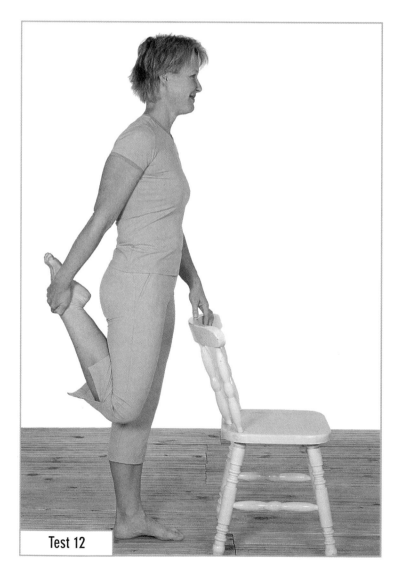

Test 12

TEST 12: QUADRICEPS
(FRONT OF THIGHS)

Stand holding onto the back of a chair with your left arm. Take your right foot in your right hand and pull it toward your right buttock. Keep your knees in line with each other and the abdominals activated so that the torso is lengthened. If you feel a stretch into the front of the thigh your quadriceps are probably tight. If you feel a stretch into the front of your groin, your hip flexors may need a good stretch too.

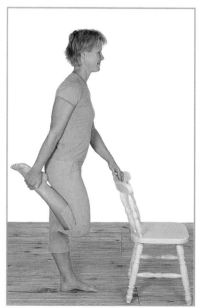

TEST 13: HIPS

Sit on a table so that your legs hang off the edge, with your feet directly underneath your knees. Keeping your right knee exactly where it is (that is, in front of the right hip), raise the right lower leg sideways to the right as high as you can without changing the position and alignment of the right knee. Now take it back to the starting point and then raise it the other way, that is, to the left, again keeping good knee alignment. Repeat with the left leg. Can you achieve a 45° angle on both sides with both legs? Raising the feet outward (right foot to right side; left foot to left side) tests tightness in the external rotators of the hip and, at the same time, the strength of your hip internal rotators. Doing the reverse (right foot to left side; left foot to right side) tests tightness in the internal rotators of the hip and the strength of your hip external rotators.

The lying torso twist (see p52) and the butterfly (see p68) will address the tightness of the external and internal rotators respectively. Over time, simply stretching these muscles will restore balance, although it would be ideal to also strengthen those muscles that appear to be weak.

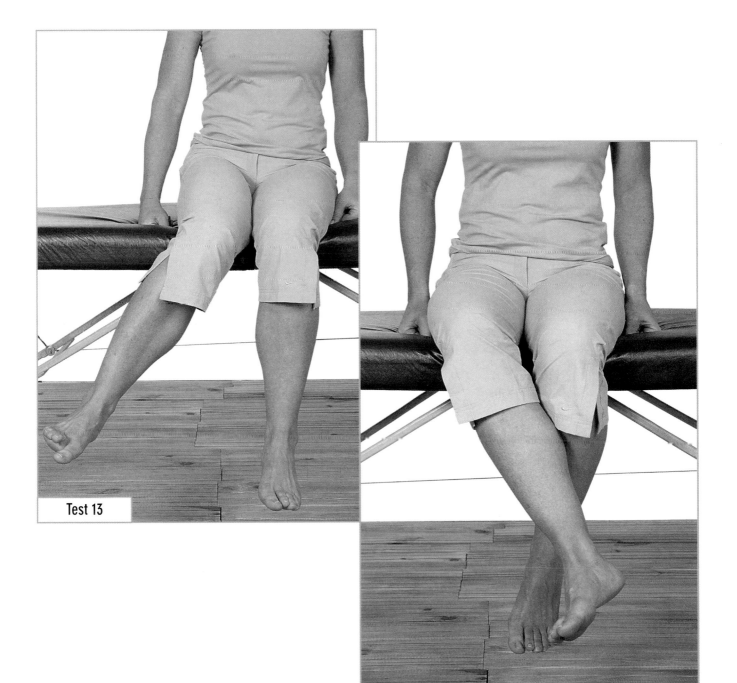

Test 13

TEST 14: HIP FLEXORS (FRONT OF HIP) AND GLUTEALS (BUTTOCKS)

Lie on the floor with both legs together and straight, knees facing the ceiling. Raise your right knee and hug it in with both hands as close to your chest as possible, without allowing your pubic bone to roll backward toward the chest (keep the buttocks firmly on the floor). The left leg should remain straight and on the floor. Repeat on the other side.

If the straight leg came off the floor, you probably have a tight hip flexor on that side. If the straight leg not only lifts off the floor, but also swings out to the side this may indicate tight external rotators of the hip as well.

If you were unable to get the knee of the bent leg close to your chest without feeling a tightness in the buttocks on that side, the gluteals of the bent leg may be tight and will require some stretching.

If you know yourself to be very inflexible, you could perform this test by bending the opposite leg ⋆, instead of keeping it straight on the floor. The need to use this position, in itself, indicates a need for stretching.

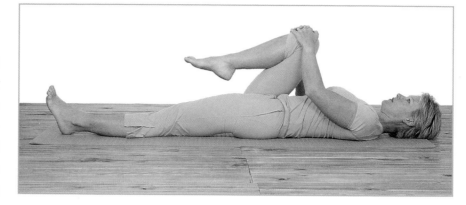

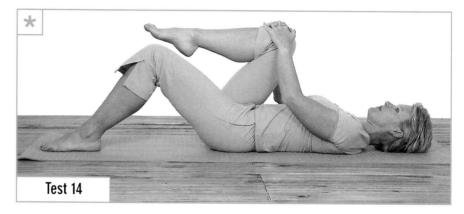

Test 14

TEST 15: CALVES 1

Stand facing a wall or behind a chair, about one pace away, feet hip distance apart. Step forward, keeping your hips square and your foot in line with your hip and put your hands on the back of the chair or palms flat against the wall. The front knee is bent, the back knee is straight, with both heels pressed down into the floor. Repeat on the other side.

Do you feel tightness in the calf muscle of the back leg (would you rate the stretch as greater than 5 on a scale of 1–10), or are you unable to keep your back heel down on the floor? If so, include stretches for the gastrocnemius muscle.

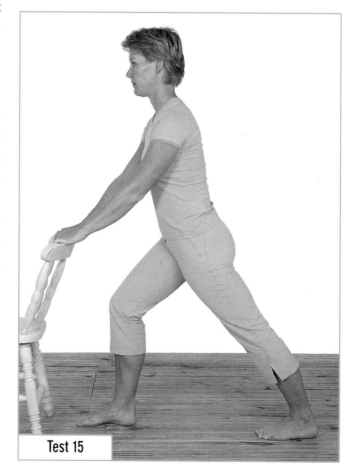

Test 15

TEST 16: CALVES 2

Do the same as with the previous stretch, but this time bring the back leg slightly closer to the front one and bend both legs.

If you feel tightness in the calf muscle of the back leg (generally more toward the ankle, and with a rating greater than 5 on a scale of 1–10), or if you are unable to keep your back heel down on the ground, you will need to add stretches for the soleus muscle to your programme.

TEST 17: SHINS

Sit on the floor, straighten your legs and point your feet (like a ballet dancer), keeping your toes directly in front of your ankles, not pointing inward (as shown in the small inset photograph ✱).

Are you able to come anywhere close to touching the floor with your toes, or can you at least get your feet and toes parallel to the floor? If you are unable to do so, this may indicate tightness in one or all the muscles that flex the foot (tibialis anterior, extensor digitorum longus, and the extensor hallucis longus muscle).

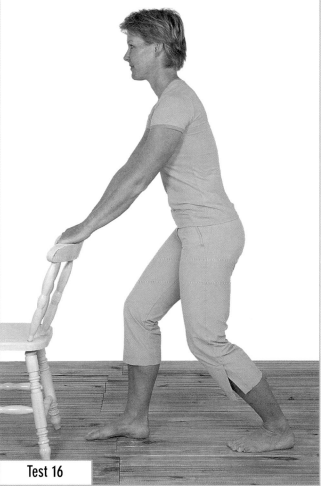

Test 16

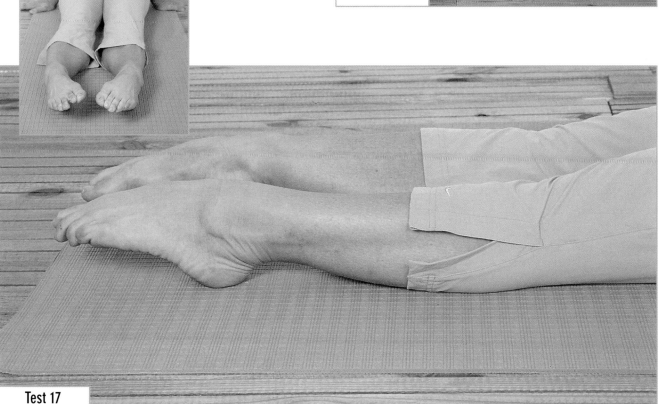

Test 17

The Menu

Each stretch on this menu is identified as either a compound or isolation stretch. Compound stretches are great time savers because they significantly stretch more than one muscle at a time, while isolation stretches are very specific and may be better if you need to target a particular muscle group.

Be sure to warm up first, perform your stretches gradually, cautiously, and in a controlled manner and to breathe normally throughout execution. Try to relax your body while in the stretches, holding each one ultimately for 60 to 90 seconds.

JOINT MOBILIZATION

Before stretching the muscles around a particular joint, it is a good idea to mobilize the joint itself by taking it through its range of motion (not necessarily the full range, but as much as is comfortable). This can be done with any activity or sport, the movements of which will lubricate the joints, allowing for easy post-workout stretching. Alternatively, you can mobilize the joints with specific exercises.

A few mobilization exercises are given before the stretches in each section.

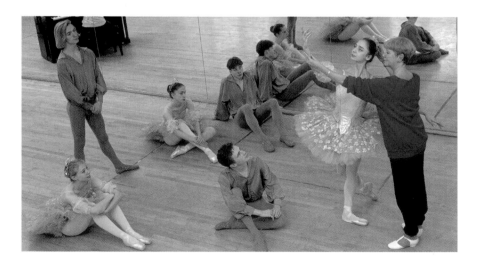

Stretching regularly will result in longer, leaner-looking muscles, giving the visual effect of being taller and slimmer.

TRUNK (FRONT) ABDOMINALS

Mobilization

TORSO REACH

Standing with your feet apart, stretch your arms up to the ceiling and then slightly further back until you feel a stretch in the abdominals. Now swing your arms down, tucking your head down and bending your knees as you do so. Let the momentum carry your arms past your body and behind your back as high as feels comfortable. Repeat five to eight times.

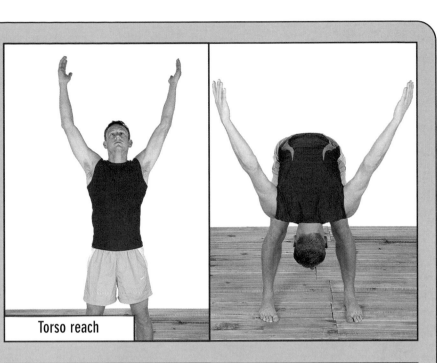

Torso reach

TORSO ROLL

Standing with your hands on your hips, gently roll your torso to the front, side, back and side again, keeping your hips still and your chest facing the front. Repeat three times before changing direction.

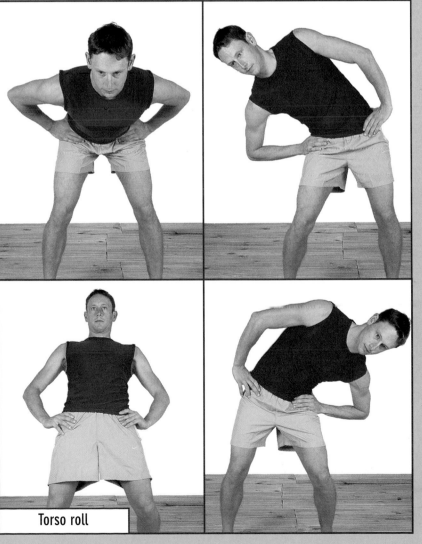

Torso roll

1a. Cobra

Type of Stretch: isolation

Main Muscle: rectus abdominus

Stretch: Lie on the floor with your hands in front of your shoulders, elbows bent and palms facing down. Breathe out as you slowly lift your torso off the ground until you reach an angle of about 45°. Attempt to push your ribcage toward the wall you are facing, until you feel a stretch across the abdominals. Relax your chest and shoulders and breathe out as you lower your chest to the floor again.

What to look out for: Be careful not to raise yourself too high off the ground, since you may compress the discs of the lumbar spine. Instead, attempt to lengthen your spine as you lift diagonally upward, as though aiming for the place where the ceiling and wall join, rather than straight up to the ceiling.

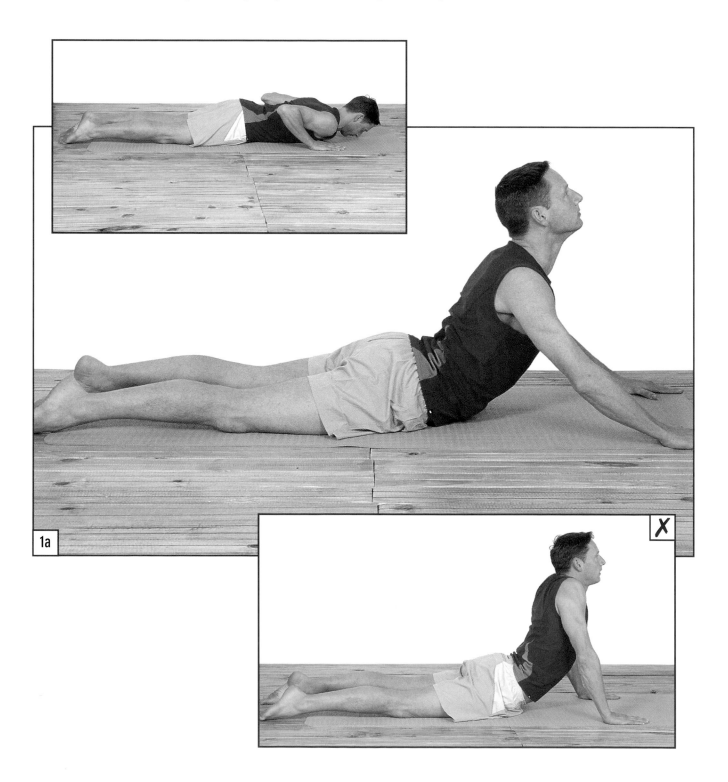

1a

X

1b. Kneeling back bend

Type of Stretch: compound

Main Muscles: abdominals, iliopsoas (hip flexors)

Stretch: Kneel on the floor with your legs hip distance apart and place your hands (fingers pointing downward) on your lower back (back of the pelvis). Lengthen your spine and then slowly lean backward, allowing your hips to move forward slightly. Look up as you move backward, but try not to let your head drop back between the shoulders. This stretch should be felt in the abdominals and across the front of the hips. Slowly bring yourself back up again. You may not be able to hold this stretch all that long, so aim for a 30- rather than 90-second stretch.

What to look out for: Keeping the spine lengthened while in this position reduces the chances of compression in the lumbar spine. Try to think of leaning back toward the wall behind you, rather than down toward the floor behind you.

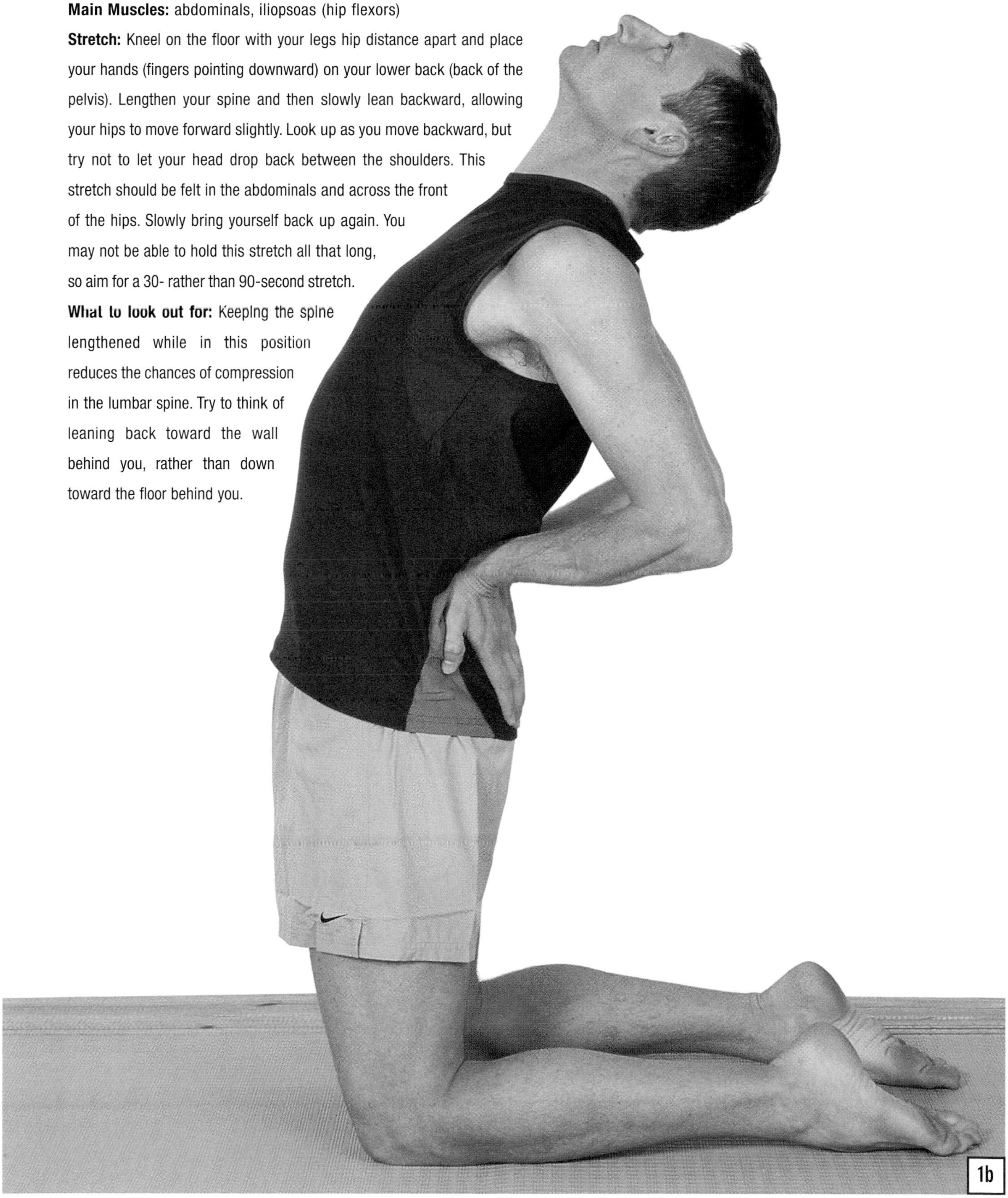

1b

2. Elevated back bend

Type of Stretch: compound

Main Muscles: abdominals, iliopsoas (hip flexors)

Stretch: Lie on your back and place two pillows or cushions under your sacrum – which is the area below your lumbar spine and above your coccyx bone. This should raise your pelvis about 10cm (4in) off the floor – just enough for you to feel a mild stretch into the abdominal area. Keep your legs straight and together. If you want to increase the stretch, you can take your arms overhead. If you experience lower back pain when doing this, then rather keep your hands at your sides.

What to look out for: Relaxing your legs in this stretch can destabilize the pelvis, which may lead to back compression and pain. It is better to stabilize the torso and pelvis by consciously tensing the thighs and flexing the feet.

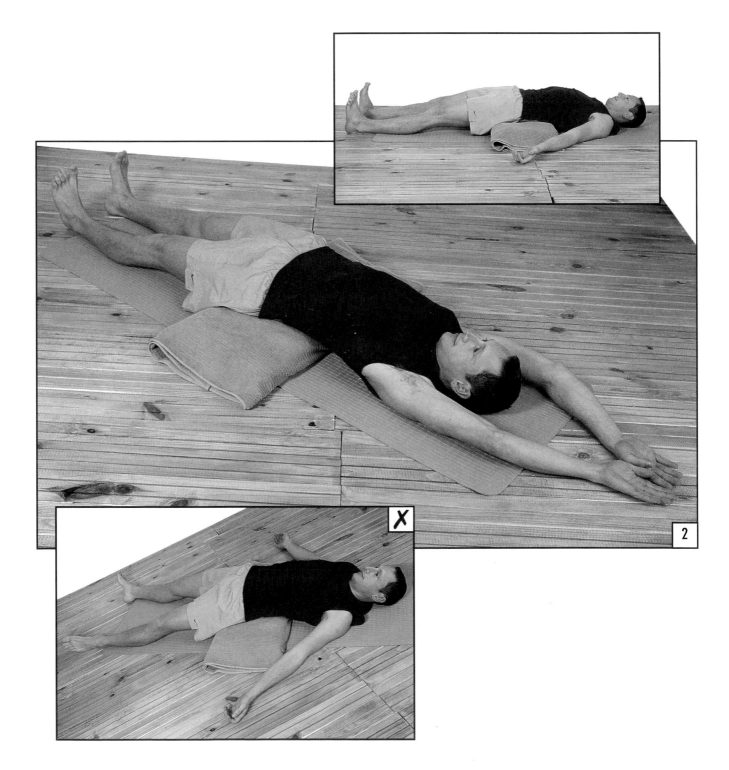

3a. Standing side stretch

Type of Stretch: compound

Main Muscles: obliques, quadratus lumborum (lower back), latissimus dorsi (mid back), teres major (mid/upper back), triceps

Stretch: Stand with your hands clasped above your head, elbows extended and palms facing away from your head. Place your feet fairly wide apart for stability and keep your navel pulled toward your spine to support the lower back. Slowly lean over to the right, stretching your hands as far as they can go. Repeat on the other side.

What to look out for: Aim to lengthen your body sideways while performing this stretch. Ensure that your chest and shoulders face forward, with the top arm directly over your top ear (not in front or behind it).

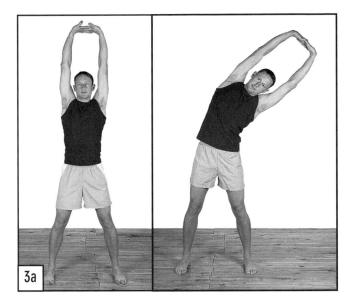

3b. Seated side stretch

Type of Stretch: compound

Main Muscles: obliques, quadratus lumborum (lower back), latissimus dorsi (mid back) and teres major (mid and upper back), as well as those targeted in the stride stretch (*see p79*), namely the leg adductors, which pull the legs together (adductor magnus, brevis and longus of the inner thigh, as well as the pectineus, which lies in front of the pubis) and the hamstrings.

Stretch: Sit on the floor with your legs straight and opened as wide as you comfortably can. Ensure that you are sitting forward on your sitting bones (ischiopubic ramus – *see glossary*) with your pelvis in neutral alignment and that you are not sitting back on the flesh of your buttocks. If your hips are tight, sit on a firm cushion or folded towel to raise them slightly. With your left hand placed on the floor, take your right arm up until it is above your head and next to your right ear. Keeping your chest facing the front, both buttocks firmly on the ground and your legs straight (with knees facing the ceiling), slowly stretch your right hand, arm and side of the body over toward the left until you feel a stretch along the right-hand side of your torso. Come up and repeat on the other side. If you are very tight in the inner thighs and find it awkward to sit with your legs open, you can do this same stretch while sitting cross-legged. Just be sure to change legs each time you do this stretch.

What to look out for: Do not allow the right buttock to come off the floor as you stretch toward the left (and vice versa when stretching toward the right), as it will minimize the stretch. Be sure to maintain neutral curvature of the spine throughout this stretch. Try to lengthen your spine and think of stretching to the top of the opposite wall as you lean over to the side.

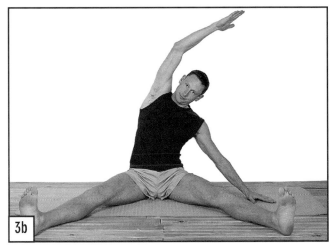

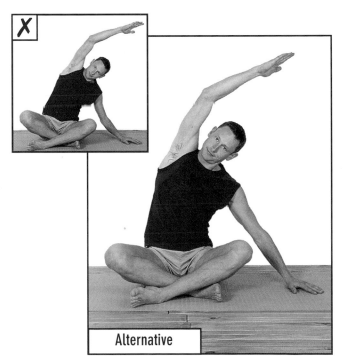

Alternative

3c. Kneeling side stretch (advanced)

Type of Stretch: compound

Main Muscles: obliques, quadratus lumborum (lower back), latissimus dorsi (mid back), teres major (mid/upper back)

Stretch: Kneel on your left leg. Extend your right leg to the side. It should be straight. Run your right hand down your right leg until you reach a point where you start to feel the stretch across the left side of your body. Hold onto your leg with this arm and slowly raise your left arm overhead. Bring your arm over so that your left hand points in the same direction as the right foot, palm down.

If you can, lower the toes of your right foot until they almost touch the floor (this will increase the stretch). Repeat on the other side.

What to look out for: As with the standing side stretch, lengthen your body sideways and ensure that your chest and shoulders face forward, with the top arm directly over your top ear. The same applies to the torso; do not allow it to lean backward – it should be directly over the extended leg – not in front of, or behind it.

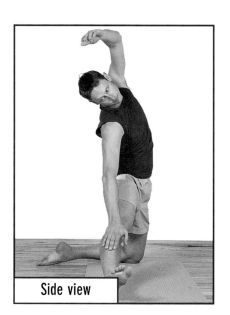

Side view

3c

CHEST

MOBILIZATION

CHEST OPENER

Stand with your arms midway between hip and shoulder height. Gently swing your arms forward and then away from your chest. Repeat five to eight times.

ARC

This exercise takes the arms and shoulders through their full range of movement and offers an effective combination of chest and shoulder work.

Sit on a stool and take the ends of a rope or strap in each hand, holding it taut in front of you. Slowly raise your arms, moving in an arc overhead to the back of the body, keeping the elbows straight, and touching the rope or strap to the buttocks at the end of the movement. Then bring them back to the front again. This exercise needs to be slow and controlled, because your shoulders are vulnerable in the third quarter of this arc. If your shoulders are very tight, you'll need to hold the rope in a wide grip to enable you to take the arms behind you. As you become looser, try and move your hands closer toward one another.

What to look out for: Do not allow your ribs to stick out, or your back to arch as you take the arms behind you; rather try to draw the front of your ribs back toward your spine. This will lengthen the spine and increase the stretch.

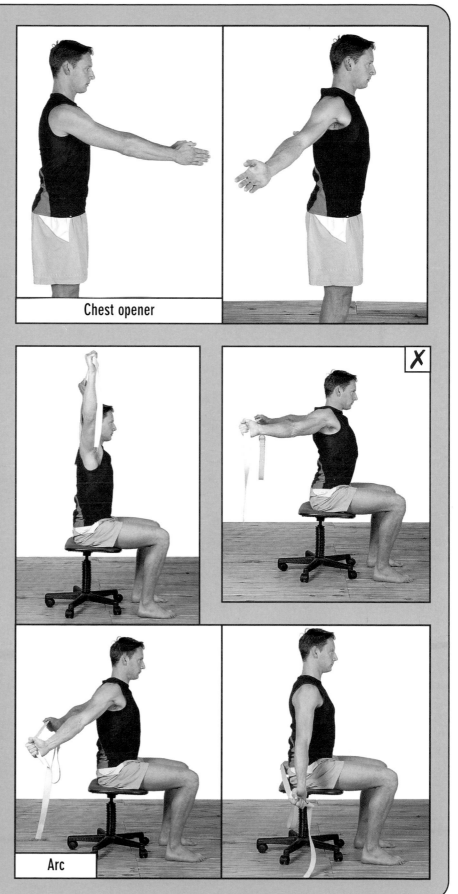

Chest opener

Arc

4a. Bent-arm wall stretch

Type of Stretch: isolation

Main Muscle: pectoralis major

Stretch: Stand next to a wall with your right elbow bent to make an angle of 90° and your palm flat against the wall. Your elbow should be at the same height as your shoulder. Step forward onto your right foot so that your right elbow is now behind you and the stretch is felt across your chest. Ensure that your hips and shoulders remain facing the front and your navel is pulled toward your spine to keep the alignment of the spine neutral (*see pelvic tilt pp27 and 87*). Repeat on the left.

What to look out for: Keep your shoulders depressed and avoid turning your torso toward the side you are stretching. Keep your navel pulled in toward your spine to avoid compression in the lumbar spine.

4b. Doorway stretch

Type of Stretch: compound

Main Muscles: pectoralis major and minor

Stretch: Stand in a doorway with your elbows, at the same height as your shoulders and bent at a 90° angle, placed on either side of you against the doorframe. Keep your palms flat against the frame. Step forward onto one foot so that your elbows are now behind you and the stretch is felt across your chest. Keep your hips and shoulders facing the front, with your navel pulled to your spine, and keeping a neutral alignment of the spine.

What to look out for: Keep your shoulders depressed and avoid compressing the lower back by lengthening the spine and pulling the front of your ribs backward and downward.

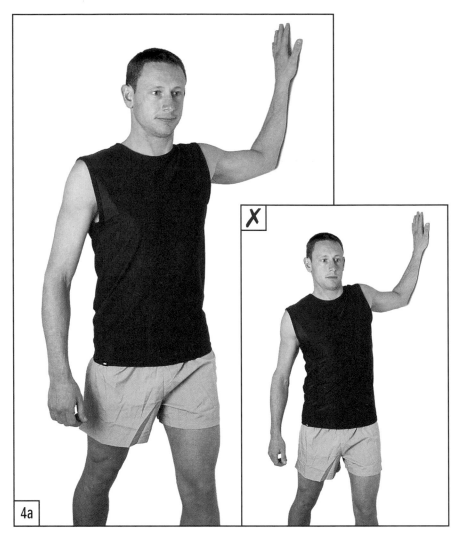

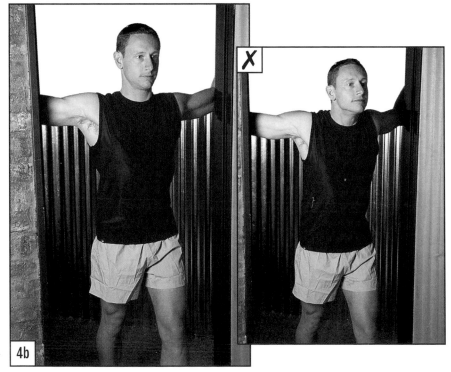

4c. Elbow squeeze
(You will need a partner for this stretch)

Type of Stretch: compound

Main Muscles: pectoralis major and minor

Stretch: Sit with your legs crossed and have some-one stand behind you, with the side of one leg placed against your spine and between your shoulder blades. Clasp your hands behind your head with your elbows bent and let your partner gently take your elbows and move them backward toward one another.

What to look out for: As with stretches 4a and 4b, keep your shoulders depressed and avoid arching the lower back by lengthening the spine and pulling the front of your ribs both backward and downward during this stretch. Caution: your partner must be very slow and gentle with the elbow movement, because this can be a very powerful stretch.

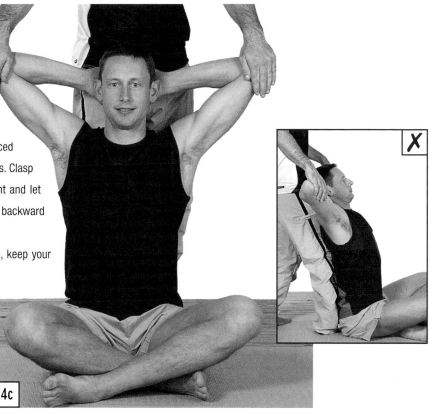

5. Lying chest opener

Type of Stretch: isolation

Main Muscle: pectoralis major

Stretch: Lie on your back, arms by your side, on a narrow bench. Bend your knees and put your feet on the bench. Your feet should be close to your buttocks to ensure that your back is supported through the stretch. Keeping your arms straight, raise them above your chest until your hands are above your nipples, palms facing one another. Slowly open your arms out to the sides of your body, bending the elbows slightly. Take your arms as far back as they will go without forcing them. You should feel a stretch across the chest.

If you don't have a narrow bench, you can lie on a bed, with your head in a corner so that your arms and elbows will be free to stretch over the sides.

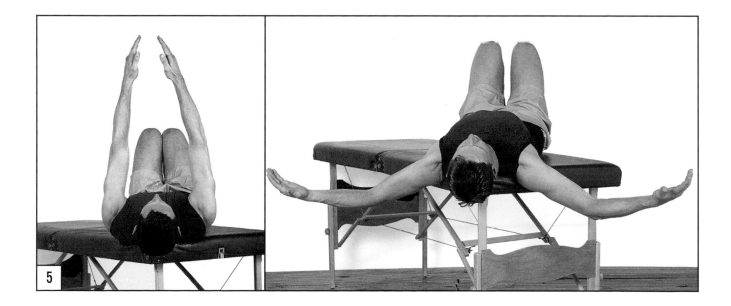

6. Hand clasp

Type of Stretch: compound

Main Muscles: pectoralis major and minor

Stretch: Stand with your feet hip distance apart and take your arms behind your back, clasping them together with palms facing each other. Roll your shoulders outward and try to cross your little fingers, as opposed to your thumbs. This will ensure that the chest is opened up for an effective stretch.

What to look out for: Avoid arching your back and sticking your ribs out during this stretch; rather, bring your ribs backward and downward and pull your navel to your spine, lengthening the spine at the same time.

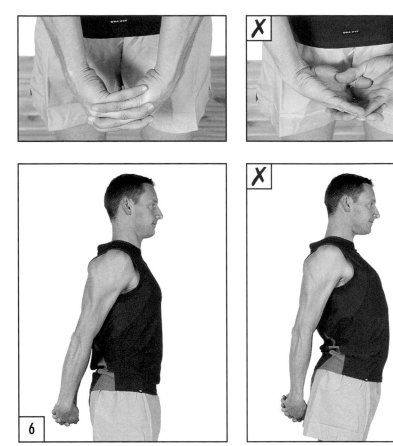

7. Chest press

Type of Stretch: isolation (you will need a partner for this one)

Main Muscle: pectoralis minor

Stretch: Lie on your back on the floor with your arms at your sides, palms facing upward. Have someone kneel at your head and cup the front of your shoulders with their hands, so that they are pushing down on your shoulders from above. You should feel a good stretch across the front of the shoulders and into the chest. To increase this stretch, place a rolled-up towel along the length of your spine. This will open up the chest further.

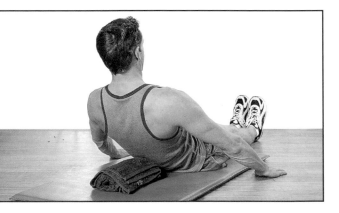

TRUNK (BACK) LOWER AND MIDDLE BACK

Mobilization

CAT STRETCH

Kneel on all fours, with your hands directly underneath your shoulders and your knees directly underneath your hips. Keep your neck in line with your spine, that is, with your face toward the floor.

Slowly arch your back, dropping your stomach toward the floor until your back is concave, but not excessively so.

Now do the reverse, rounding your back until it is convex. Repeat five to eight times.

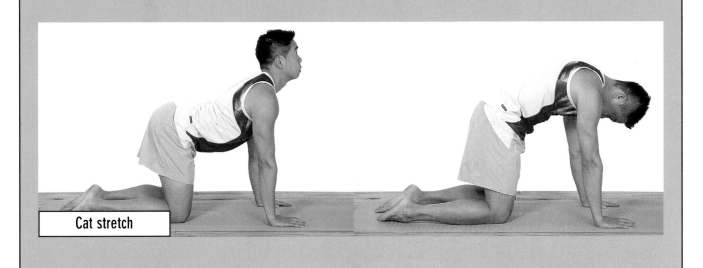

Cat stretch

TORSO SWING

Stand with your legs slightly apart and your hands loosely at your sides. Swing your torso lightly to the right with your hips moving freely, allowing your left arm to cross in front of your body and your right arm to cross behind your back. Now do the same to the left side. Repeat four or five times to each side.

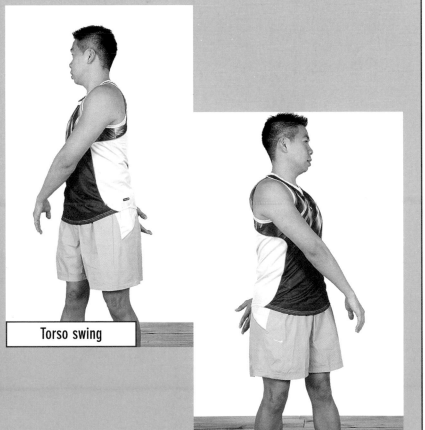

Torso swing

8. Child pose (a yoga term)

Type of Stretch: isolation

Main Muscle: erector spinae

Stretch: Sit back on your feet. Slowly lean forward until your head rests on the floor in front of your knees, resting on the top of your forehead (above your hairline). Rest your hands on the floor and at your sides, with the palms facing upward. In this position, your spine should be well rounded.

What to look out for: Avoid arching and thus compressing the neck when the head is resting on the floor; rather tuck in your chin toward your chest, keeping the neck in line with the spine.

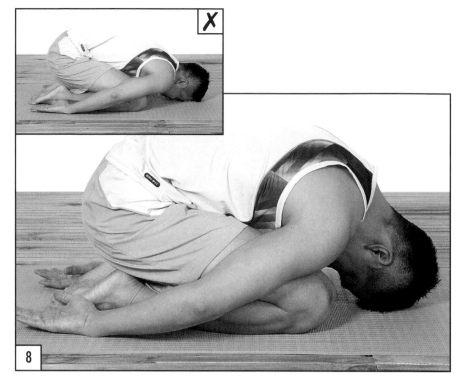

9. Tree hug

Type of Stretch: compound

Main Muscles: erector spinae, rhomboids, trapezius

Stretch: Stand with the feet approximately hip distance apart and clasp your hands in front of your body at chest height. Bend your knees, curl your pelvis upward toward your head and your head down toward your pelvis as you round the back into a C-shape.

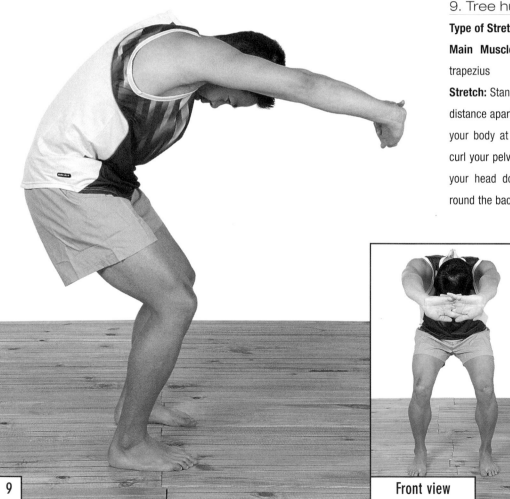

Front view

10. Forward hanging stretch

Type of Stretch: compound

Main Muscles: erector spinae, hamstrings, and calf muscles

Stretch: Stand with your feet shoulder width apart, hands at your sides and your knees soft (lightly bent). Tuck your chin in toward your chest and slowly drop your torso toward the floor, rolling one vertebra at a time so that the spine is curved throughout the forward movement. Go as far as you can, stopping when you feel a stretch in the back of your legs, back or calves (or all three). If you are able to get that far, rest your hands on the floor in front of you, palms facing down and fingers pointing forward. If you are unable to touch the floor, place your hands on a chair, box or cushions stacked in front of your feet. This will provide your back with support while you are in the stretch.

What to look out for: Avoid looking up while performing this stretch, as it compresses the neck; keep your chin tucked in toward your chest. You may feel a stretch into your back when you do this. However, if it is not severe, try and stay with this position, because you will also be stretching the muscles in the back of your neck. Avoid straightening your knee joints, unless you are able to touch the floor, since this will increase the stretch into your hamstrings and back.

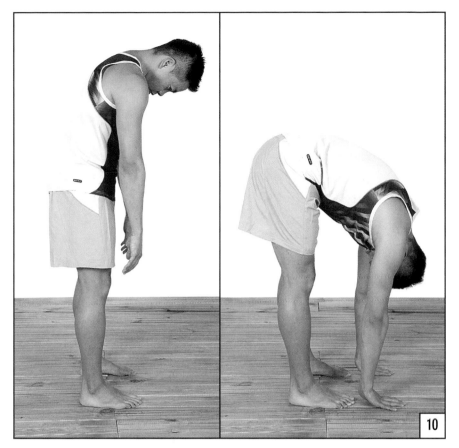

10

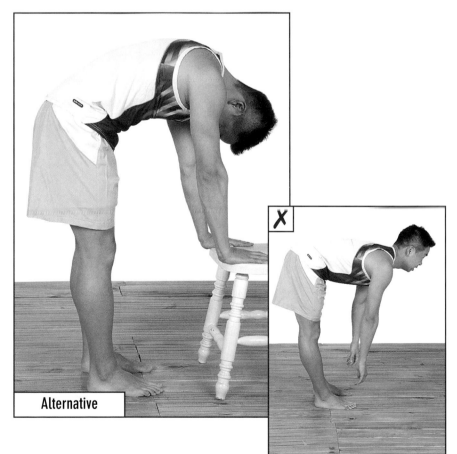

Alternative

11. Lying torso twist

Type of Stretch: compound

Main Muscles: gluteals, deep external rotators of hips (piriformis, gemellus superior and inferior, obturator externus and internus, quadratus femoris), lower aspect of erector spinae, obliques, latissimus dorsi, quadratus lumborum

Stretch: Lie on your back with your legs straight and your arms out to the sides in a straight line with your shoulders, palms down. Bend your right leg and pull it in toward your chest, keeping your left leg straight and on the ground. Leaving your right hand on the floor, use your left hand to take your right knee gently over toward the left until it touches the floor, or until you feel a stretch pulling across your back. Ensure that your torso continues to face the ceiling so that the right shoulder stays on the floor (this sounds easier than it is). If your knee does not touch the floor, place a pillow underneath it to support the weight of the leg. However, if the pillow is too high it will diminish the stretch. If your knee touches the floor easily enough, you can try extending your leg to intensify the stretch (this adds more weight into the stretch). Come out of this stretch slowly before repeating on the other side.

What to look out for: Twists can be very intense stretches, so avoid moving into and out of them too quickly. Also, don't push the stretch further than feels comfortable and make sure you breathe throughout the stretch, since twists can feel constrictive if not done correctly.

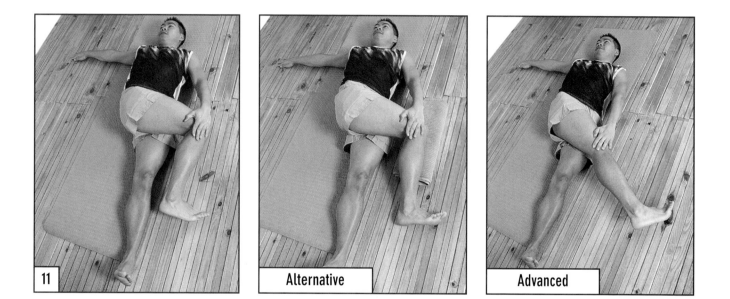

11 | Alternative | Advanced

12a. The frog stretch

Type of Stretch: compound

Main Muscles: latissimus dorsi, teres major, rhomboids, mid-trapezius and posterior deltoid

Stretch: Sit back on your feet with your toes together and your knees apart. Slowly lower your torso toward the floor between your knees, resting on the top of your forehead (on your hairline). Now extend your arms in front of you on the floor, palms down. Keep your elbows straight and off the ground while you gently push your chest toward the floor. You should feel this stretch into your back and the sides of your armpits.

What to look out for: Avoid lifting your shoulders when in this stretch. Instead, visualize drawing your shoulders down your back toward the buttocks, as this action will intensify the stretch by broadening the back.

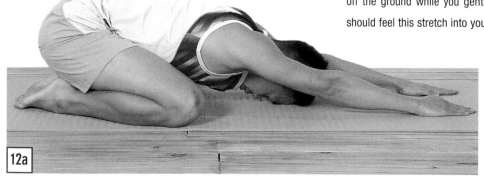

12a

12b. Standing pull-back

Type of Stretch: compound

Main Muscles: latissimus dorsi, teres major, rhomboids, mid trapezius and posterior deltoid

Stretch: With your feet hip distance apart, stand facing the edge of an open door, far enough away from the handles so that when you place your hands on the handles on each side of the door and then lean backward until your arms are straight, your body will form a V-shape, with your feet forward of your hips, on a diagonal line. Bend your knees and, keeping a flat back, pull away from the door. You should feel the stretch in your back. This stretch can also be performed by pulling off the back of a chair – as long as someone is sitting in it for the duration of the stretch!

What to look out for: Avoid arching your lower back and pushing your chest down toward the floor; rather, try to keep your back rounded (convex) while in this position.

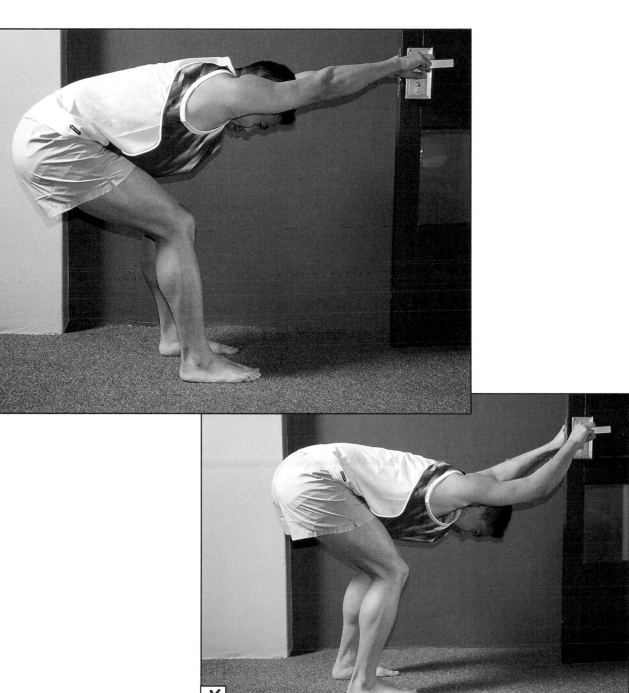

12b

X

UPPER BACK

Mobilization

UPPER SPINE ROLL

Tuck your chin in toward your chest and gently roll your head down toward your waist, rounding your upper back as much as possible. Roll back up again and finish off the movement by lifting your chest toward the ceiling (let your head tilt backward). Repeat five to eight times.

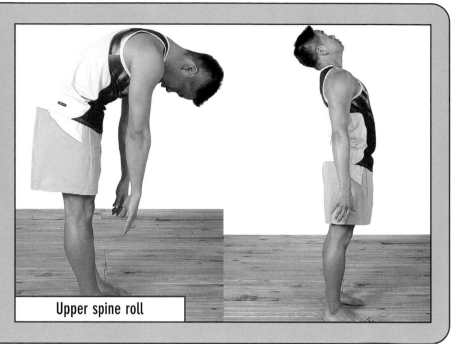

Upper spine roll

13a. Arm-across-chest

Type of Stretch: compound

Main Muscles: rhomboids and middle trapezius

Stretch: Stand in a comfortable position and take hold of your right wrist with your left hand, drawing it across your chest at shoulder height. Keep your chest and hips facing the front as you gently pull the arm as far to the left as possible. Repeat on the other side.

What to look out for: Avoid raising the shoulder of your working arm, as this action will diminish the stretch (which should be felt across the upper back). Also avoid turning the chest toward the direction in which the arm is being pulled, for the same reason.

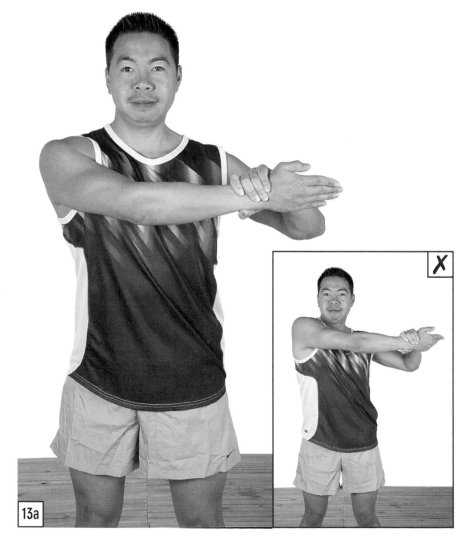

13b. Hand-over-knee

Type of Stretch: compound

Main Muscles: rhomboids and middle trapezius

Stretch: Sit on a bench with your legs shoulder width apart and your feet flat on the floor. Place each hand around the outside of the opposite knee (that is, right hand around the outside of the left knee and vice versa). Drop your head down and bend the top of your torso forward, with your spine rounded, as you pull your knees apart. You should feel this stretch between your shoulder blades. Repeat with hands crossed the other way (left over right or vice versa).

What to look out for: Avoid raising your shoulders during this stretch. It should feel as though your shoulder blades are being drawn down toward your buttocks.

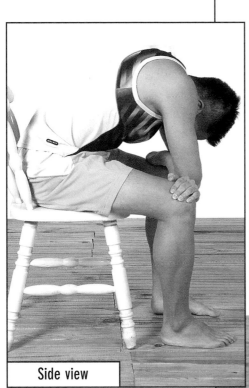

Side view

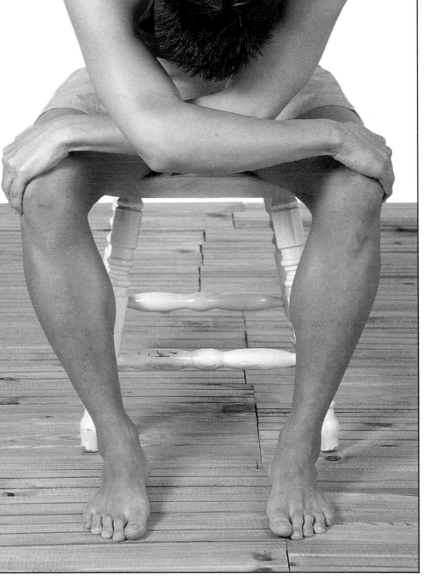

13b

14. Snake

Type of Stretch: compound

Main Muscles: trapezius (especially mid and lower), posterior deltoid, rhomboids, infraspinatus, teres major and minor, subscapularis

Stretch: Sit or stand and bend your left arm, bringing the elbow in front of your chest and up at nipple height. Your left hand should be directly above your left elbow. Now bring your right hand in front of your chest and cross your right elbow over your left arm, fitting the elbow of your right arm as far over the crook of your left elbow as possible. Join your hands and slowly raise your elbows slightly, until you feel a stretch pulling across your upper back, below your neck, and back of the armpit. Repeat on the other side.

If you are unable to cross your elbows, simply take hold of your right wrist with your left hand and pull it across the front of your chest, keeping it in line with your shoulders. Ensure that your chest remains facing the front (that is, do not swing to face the left). Repeat on the other side.

What to look out for: As with the hand-over-knee stretch, avoid raising your shoulders; rather visualize your shoulder blades being drawn down toward your buttocks.

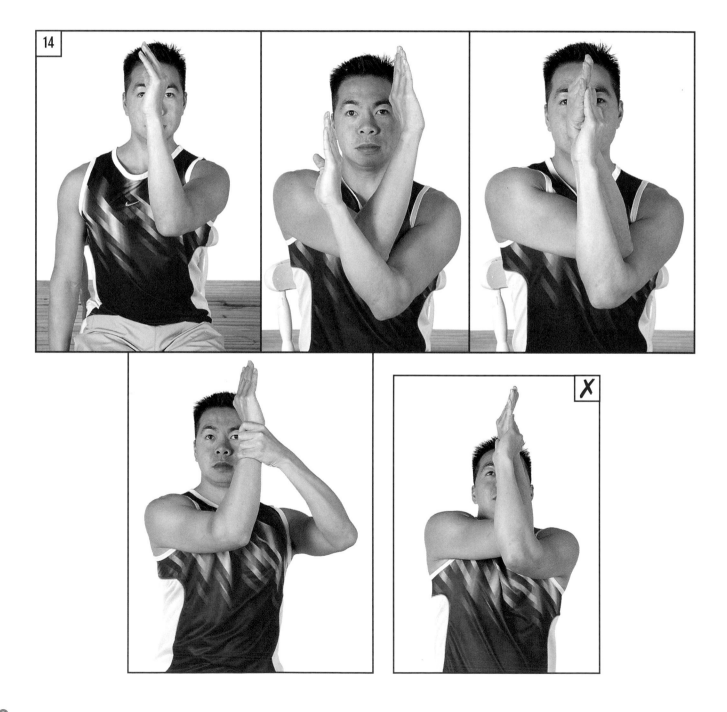

NECK

Mobilization

HEAD ROLL

Drop your head forward and roll it slowly from side to side. Look up to face the front and turn your head from side to side as far as it will comfortably go. Face the front and then slowly take your head back, allowing it to drop as far as is comfortable. Repeat the entire head roll sequence five to eight times.

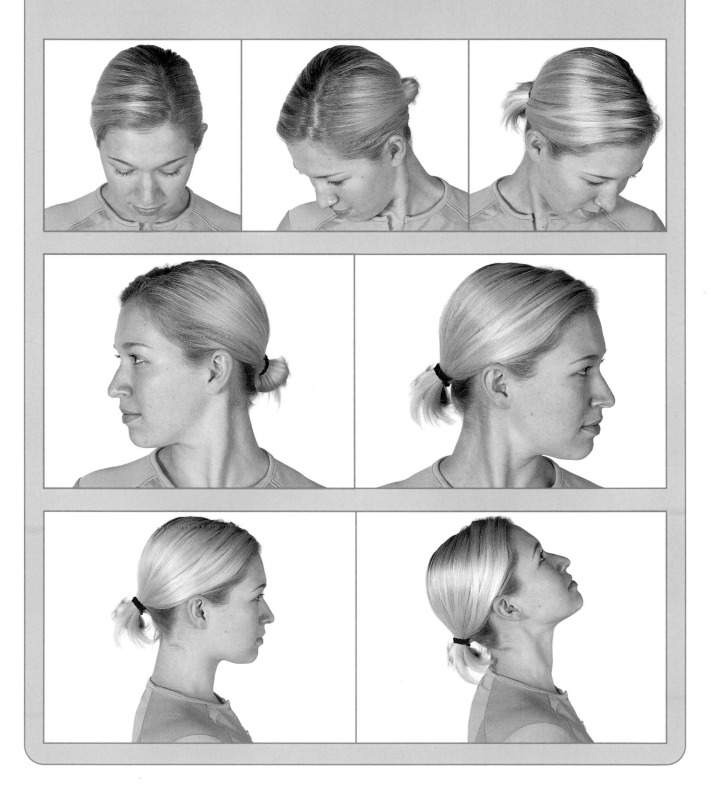

15. Seated neck stretch

Type of Stretch: compound

Main Muscles: levator scapulae, splenius, sternocleidomastoid, and the upper trapezius

Stretch: Sit or stand and bring your right hand up in front of you. Place it on the back of your skull (just behind the crown of your head). Gently pull your head down toward your chest, feeling a stretch on the back of your neck.

Face the front again and bring up your right arm on the side, again placing your hand on top of your head. Slowly drop your head to the right, bringing your right ear toward your right shoulder. You should feel the stretch on the left side of your neck.

Face the front again and then look into the right-hand corner of the room. Bring your right arm up and put it on your head, so that your elbow also points toward the right-hand corner. Slowly drop your head to look at the floor, but still over to the right. You should feel this stretch in the back of the neck, behind the left ear. Repeat the sequence on the other side, using the other hand.

What to look out for: Keep the shoulders pressed down in any neck stretch – raising them diminishes the effect of the stretch substantially.

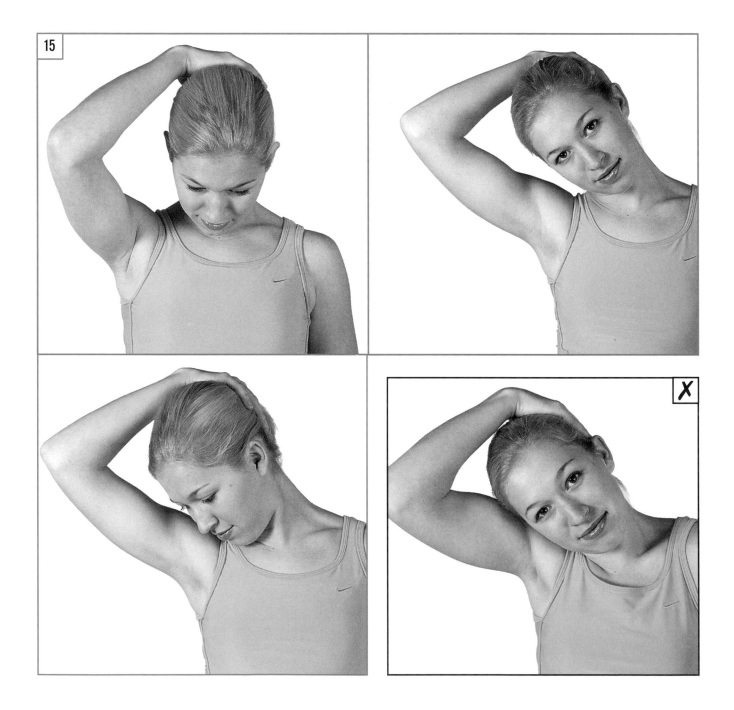

16. Lying neck stretch

Type of Stretch: compound

Main Muscles: levator scapulae, splenius, upper trapezius

Stretch: Lie on the floor on your back, with your legs straight and knees close together. Place a small towel under the base of your skull, so that it cradles the head and, keeping each end in your hands, gently lift the towel upward and forward until you feel a good stretch into the back of your neck.

What to look out for: Be gentle with your neck on this stretch, because you are stretching an area that is often very tight and thus may have limited movement.

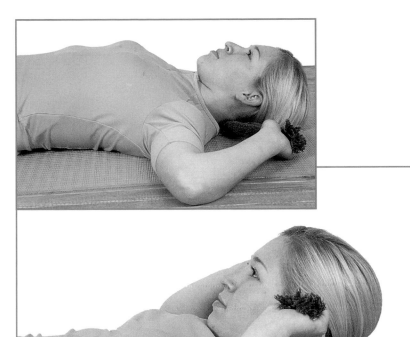

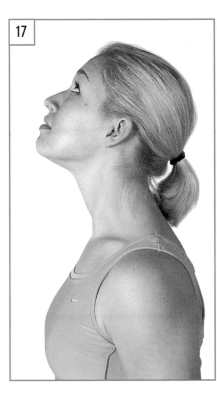

17. Throat stretch

Type of Stretch: compound

Main Muscles: sternocleidomastoid and the muscles covering the throat (sternohyoid, sternothyroid)

Stretch: Stand or sit with your navel pulled in toward your spine. With your shoulders depressed, your mouth closed and your chin jutting forward, slowly tilt your head backward until you feel a stretch down the front of your throat and neck.

What to look out for: Avoid dropping the back of the head into the shoulders, because this compresses the vertebrae in the neck. Instead, keep the movement controlled and take it only as far as feels comfortable.

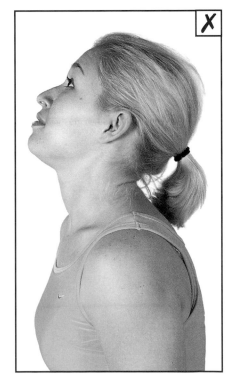

ARMS: SHOULDERS

Mobilization

ARM SWINGS

Stand with your feet comfortably apart and your arms loosely at your sides. Gently swing your right arm in a circle five times in each direction. Repeat with the left arm.

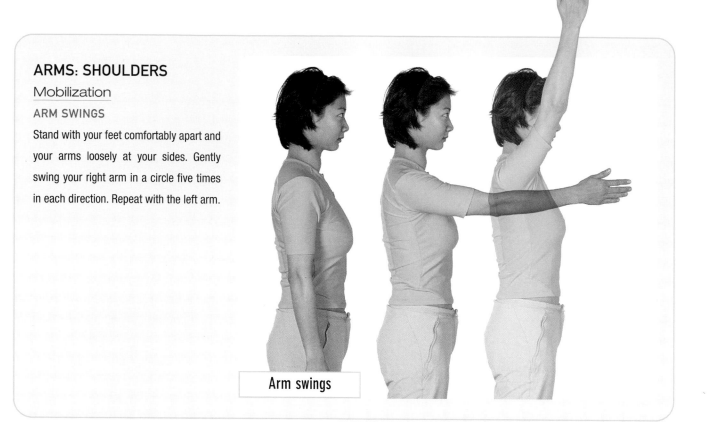

Arm swings

18. Elbow up/elbow down

Type of Stretch: compound

Main Muscles: triceps, latissimus dorsi, teres major, lower pectorals of top arm; anterior deltoid, upper pectorals of bottom arm

Stretch: Sit or stand with your spine in neutral alignment (*see pelvic tilt pp27 and 87*). Take your left arm behind your back with the palm facing away from your back and bend the elbow so that your fingers point up your spine. Stretch your right arm up to the ceiling, bend the elbow and bring the hand down, with the palm facing your back, to clasp the right hand. If your hands can't meet, take the ends of a strap or belt in each hand. Ensure that you keep your ribs tucked in and open up your chest (do not allow the shoulder of the lower arm to roll forward). Attempt to flatten the armpit of your raised arm and keep your elbow close to your ear (pointing up toward the ceiling). Your lower arm should be as close to the body as possible (try to avoid allowing a space between your waist and your elbow). Repeat on the other side.

What to look out for: As with the 'arc' stretch, do not allow your ribs to stick out, and don't allow your back to arch as you take your arms behind you. Instead, you should draw the front of your ribs back toward your spine, because this will lengthen the spine and increase the stretch.

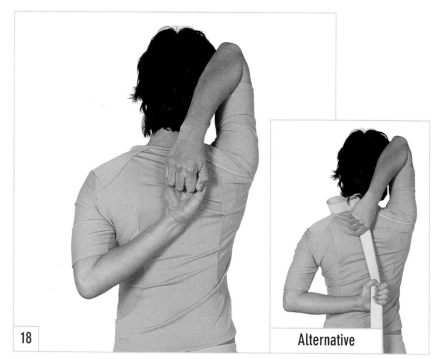

18

Alternative

19. Strap stretch

Type of Stretch: compound

Main Muscles: triceps, posterior deltoid, latissimus dorsi, teres major, lower pectorals

Stretch: Using a rope or strap, measure a loop that, when placed around your upper arms, will hold your elbows shoulder width apart. Place the loop just above your elbows (on the armpit side of the elbow) and kneel in front of a bench, about 1m (3ft) away. Grip a ball (the size of a soccer ball) or a book (placed lengthways) between your wrists. The purpose of the book or ball is to keep your hands apart, but not wider than your elbows. Rest your elbows on the edge of the bench, keeping your hands directly above your elbows. Slowly lower your torso, dropping your head between your elbows and below the level of the bench. Tuck your chin in toward your chest so that the neck is lengthened. The distance from your knees to the bench should be such that you can keep your knees directly underneath your hips. If your shoulders are very tight, make the loop bigger.

What to look out for: Avoid arching your back, which puts unnecessary pressure on your lower back and detracts from the stretch.

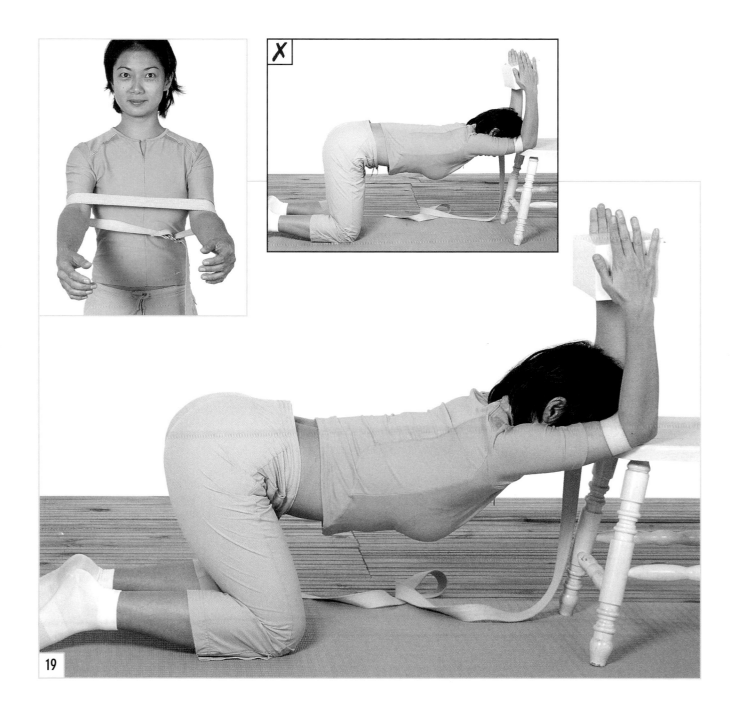

19

20. Chicken

Type of Stretch: compound

Main Muscles: teres minor, infraspinatus, posterior deltoid

Stretch: Stand with your hands behind your back, palms facing away from the body and each hand flat against the back of its corresponding hip, with elbows out to the sides. Gently pull the elbows forward until you feel a stretch behind the shoulders and into the back.

What to look out for: Keep your shoulders depressed and your navel pulled toward your spine while performing this stretch.

21. Reverse namaste

(*Namaste* is a Sanskrit word used in yoga, which means greeting. It is also a *mudra*, which means gesture – usually a symbolic one.)

Type of Stretch: compound

Main Muscles: anterior deltoids, wrist extensors

Stretch: Stand with both feet on the floor and reach your arms behind your body with your palms facing away from your body, the back of the hands flat against your back. Now bring the tips of your fingers together, turning your palms inward to face one another until you are able to place the hands palm to palm. Open up the chest by rolling the shoulders outward and attempt to work your hands as far up your back as possible (between the shoulder blades is ideal). If you are unable to touch palms and fingers, simply hold your hands behind your back – clasping each elbow in the opposite hand. You will feel this stretch into the front of your shoulders and the inside of your wrists.

What to look out for: Keep your shoulders depressed and your palms together (they tend to separate if your shoulders are tight). Also, do not allow your ribs to protrude or your lower back to arch. Instead try to draw the front of your ribs back toward your spine.

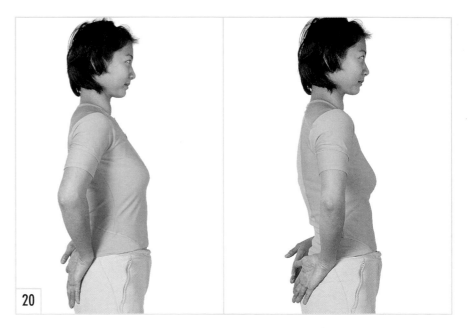

20

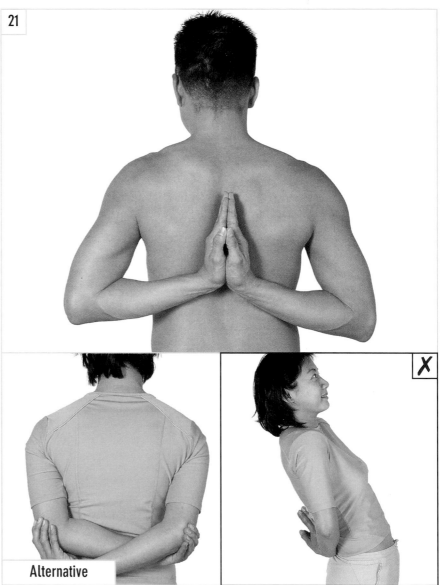

21

Alternative

X

22a. Kneeling hand clasp

Type of Stretch: compound

Main Muscles: anterior deltoids, pectorals

Stretch: Kneel on the floor, sit back on your feet and take your arms behind your back, clasping them together with palms facing each other. As with the 'hand clasp' stretch (*see p48*), roll your shoulders outward and try to cross your little fingers together (as opposed to your thumbs), because this will ensure that the chest is opened up for an effective stretch. Slowly lower your head to the floor until the top of your head rests on the ground, close to your knees, while you take your hands as high as you can.

What to look out for: Avoid lifting your shoulders. Keep them depressed and your fingers interlocked (they tend to want to separate if your shoulders are tight).

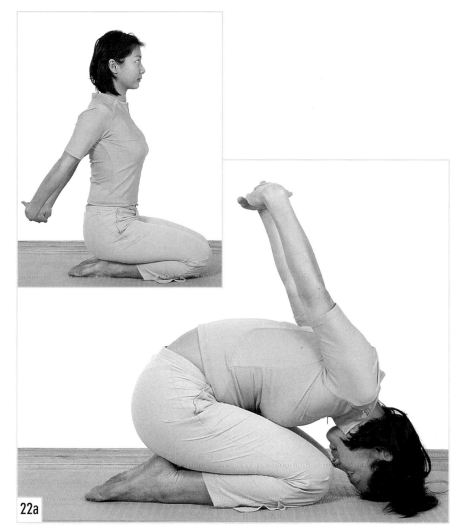

22a

22b. Straight-arm bridge

Type of Stretch: compound

Main Muscles: anterior deltoids, pectorals

Stretch: Sit on the floor with your legs straight in front of you and your hands flat on the floor behind you, fingers pointing away from your body. Keeping your elbows and knees straight, slowly raise your hips as high as you can. Keep your head in line with your neck. You should experience a stretch into the front of your shoulders.

What to look out for: Ensure that your shoulders remain depressed in order to create length in the neck (thus avoiding compression). Also keep your navel pulled toward your spine throughout this stretch.

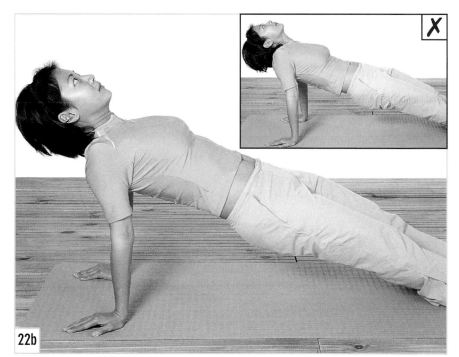

22b

ARMS AND SHOULDERS

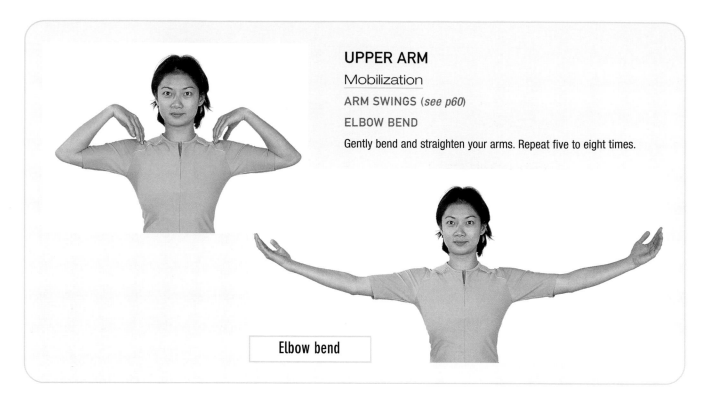

UPPER ARM

Mobilization

ARM SWINGS (*see p60*)

ELBOW BEND

Gently bend and straighten your arms. Repeat five to eight times.

Elbow bend

23. Straight-arm wall stretch

Type of Stretch: compound

Main Muscles: biceps, pectorals, anterior deltoids

Stretch: This is almost the same as the bent-arm wall stretch (*see p46*), except that this time you extend your arm so that the elbow is straight and your arm parallel to the floor. Stand next to a wall with your right arm straight and your palm flat against the wall. Your palm should be at the same height as your shoulder. Step forward onto your right foot until you feel the stretch. Now turn the arm so that the back of your hand is against the wall. Repeat on the other side.

What to look out for: Keep your shoulders depressed and avoid turning your torso toward the side you are stretching. Keep your navel pulled in toward your spine, in order to avoid compression in the lumbar spine.

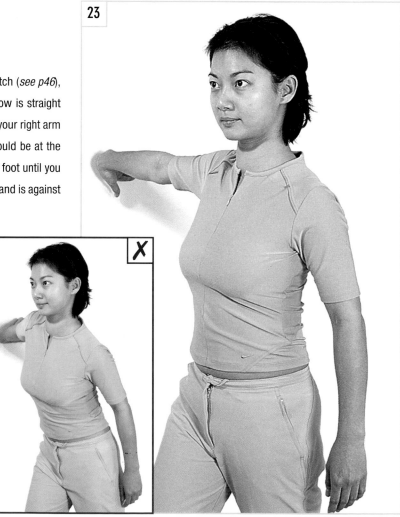

24. Elbow up

Type of Stretch: isolation

Main Muscles: triceps

Stretch: This is the same as the elbow up/elbow down stretch (*see p60*), only this time you do not use the bottom arm at all. Simply hold the top elbow with the other hand and pull it gently further down behind your head. To increase the stretch, try to keep the hand of the arm being stretched on the back of the same shoulder. Repeat on the other side.

What to look out for: As with the elbow up/elbow down stretch, do not allow your ribs to stick out, or your back to arch as you take the arm behind you. Instead, draw the front of your ribs backward toward your spine. This will lengthen the spine and increase the effectiveness of the stretch.

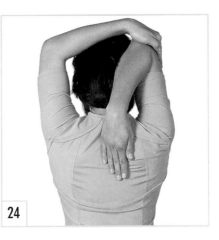

24

FOREARM AND WRIST

Mobilization

WRIST ROLL

Slowly roll your hands in a circle, moving first one way and then the other. Repeat five to eight times each way.

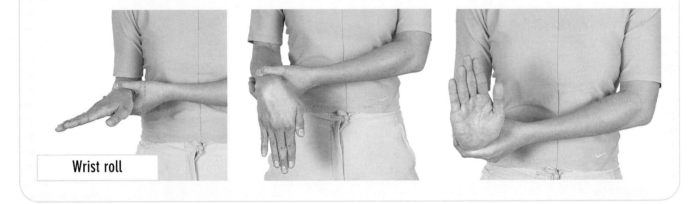

Wrist roll

25. Kneeling wrist stretch

Type of Stretch: compound

Main Muscles: wrist flexors

Stretch: Kneel on all fours, with your knees directly under your hips and your hands slightly forward of your shoulders. Your palms should be flat on the floor, fingers pointing toward your knees. Keep the elbows straight. Gently lean your body back toward your heels, until you feel a stretch into the inside of the wrists.

What to look out for: Do not stretch too fast or too hard and keep your shoulders depressed.

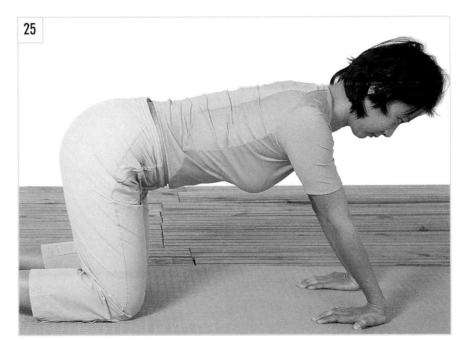

25

26. Scarecrow stretch

Type of Stretch: compound

Main Muscles: wrist extensors

Stretch: Stand with both feet on the floor and arms extended sideways so that your hands are in a direct line with your shoulders, palms facing the floor and fingers extended. Gently bend the wrists until your fingers point down toward the floor, or until you feel a stretch into the top of the wrists. For an added forearm stretch, rotate the arms inward until the tops of your wrists face forward.

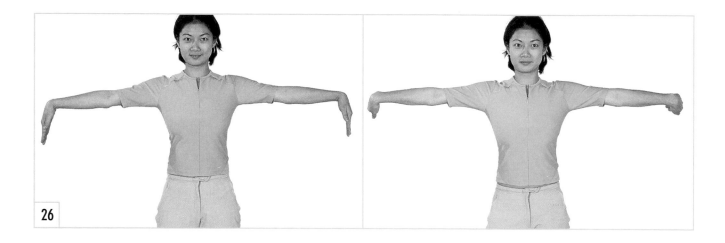

27. Hand press

Type of Stretch: compound

Main Muscles: finger flexors

Stretch: Stand or sit and press your palms together in front of your chest in a prayer position. Slide the heel of your right hand upward until it rests against the fingers of your left hand. Keeping the wrist of your left hand straight, gently push your fingers toward the left with your right hand until you feel a stretch on the underside of your fingers. Repeat on the other side.

What to look out for: Be gentle with yourself on this stretch; do not use excessive force.

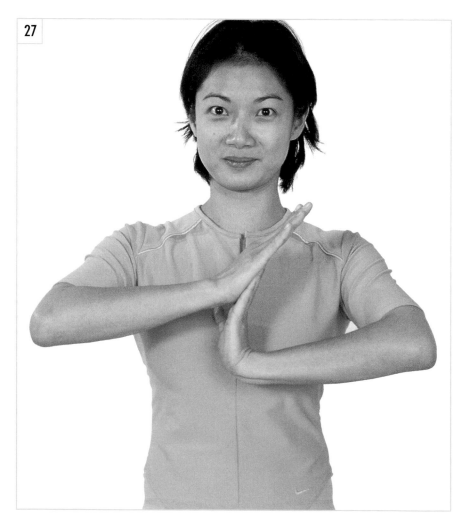

LEGS: HIPS

Mobilization

HIP ROLL

Stand on the left leg and bend your right knee, bringing it upward and moving it in a circular motion across the front of the body and then outward toward the side. Keep your hands out to the sides at shoulder height for balance. Repeat four times before reversing the direction.

Repeat, standing on the right leg.

LEG SWING

Stand on your left leg, with your hands out to the sides at shoulder height for balance. With the knee slightly bent, swing your right leg gently forward and backward, as high as you can comfortably go, but without using momentum to force it higher. Do four repetitions each way.

Now swing the leg across the front of the body, toward your left and then away from your body, toward the right-hand side, again, as high as you can comfortably go without using momentum. Again, do four repetitions each way.

Repeat, standing on the right leg.

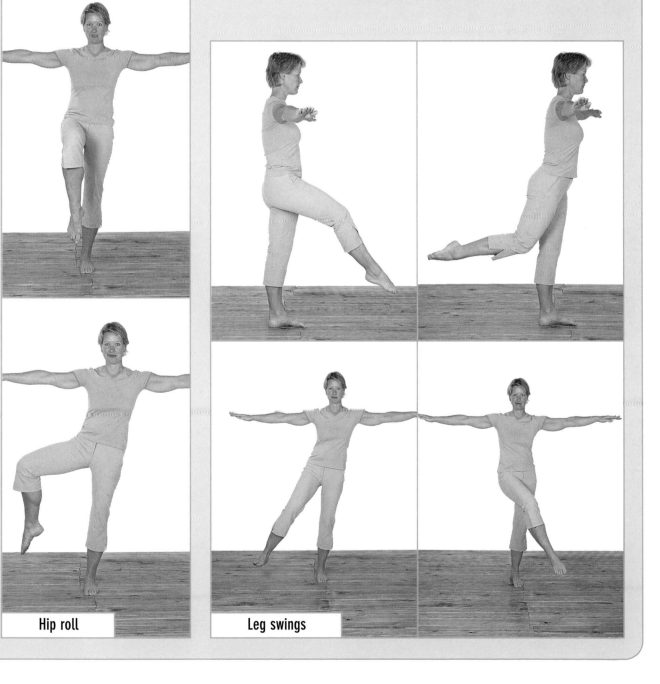

Hip roll

Leg swings

28a. Butterfly

Type of Stretch: compound

Main Muscles: the leg adductors (namely the adductor magnus, brevis and longus of the inner thigh, as well as the pectineus, which lies in front of the pubis) and the internal leg/hip rotators (tensor fasciae latae, gluteus medius and minimus, gracilis)

Stretch: Sit with your knees bent and the soles of your feet touching. Ensure that you are sitting forward on your sitting bones (*see p43 and glossary*) with your pelvis in neutral alignment, and that you are not sitting back on the flesh of your buttocks. Pull the flesh out from under your sitting bones if necessary. If your hips are tight, sit on a firm cushion or folded towel to raise them slightly. Hold your ankles with your hands. Keeping your back straight, lean forward to place your elbows on your knees, pushing them down gently. An advanced version of this can be done lying on your back. However, the abdominal muscles must be activated to ensure that your lumbar spine does not become compressed.

What to look out for: Keep your spine in neutral alignment for an optimal stretch. Avoid the tendency to round your upper and lower back, diminishing the stretch in the process.

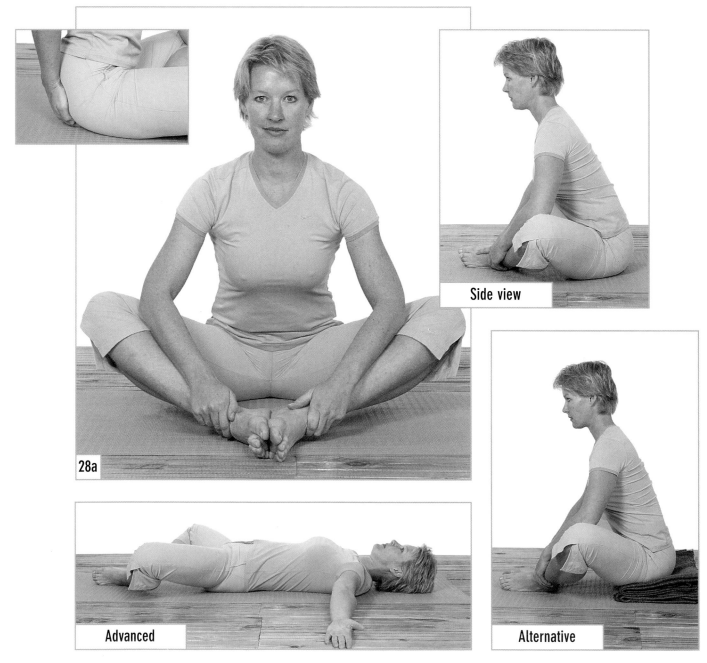

28a

Side view

Advanced

Alternative

28b. Squat stretch (plié)

Type of Stretch: compound

Main Muscles: the internal leg/hip rotators (tensor fasciae latae, gluteus medius and minimus, gracilis) and the leg adductors (namely the adductor magnus, brevis and longus of the inner thigh, as well as the pectineus, which lies in front of the pubis)

Stretch: Hold on to the back of a chair and place your feet 60–70cm (24–30in) apart, with the legs externally rotated (i.e. with your feet pointing outward on the diagonal). Ensuring that you keep your knees in line with the middle of your feet (and not rolling in front of, or behind them) and your heels on the ground throughout the stretch, slowly bend your knees and drop your bottom down toward the ground until you feel a stretch in the inner thighs and the back of the hips. You can increase this stretch by pushing your knees gently outward with your elbows.

What to look out for: Be very aware of keeping your knees in line with your middle toes because, if you have a tendency to roll them inward, you may put unnecessary strain on the inside of the knee joint.

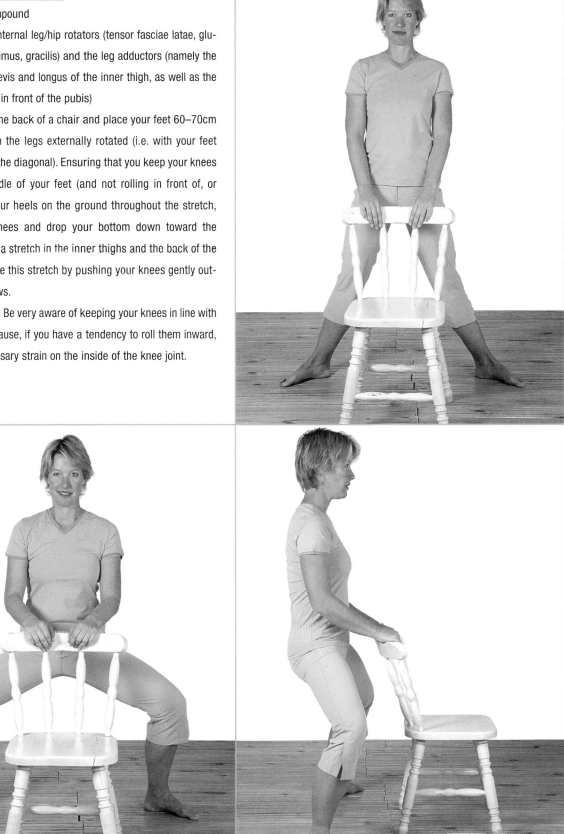

26b

Side view

29a. Foot-over-knee

Type of Stretch: compound

Main Muscles: gluteus maximus, hamstrings (to a lesser degree)

Stretch: Lie on your back with your left leg bent, foot flat on the floor. Place your right foot onto your left knee with the foot flexed. Clasp your left knee in your arms (you'll need to pass your right arm between your legs) and pull it upward toward your chest. If you find it difficult to keep your head down on the floor, put a pillow or cushion underneath it. Try to relax the upper body and breathe through this stretch. This stretch will be felt in the buttock of the right leg. Repeat on the other side.

If you find it more comfortable, you could perform this stretch against a wall, so that the arms are free. Lie on your back as before, with your buttocks toward a wall. Place your left foot against the wall, so that your lower leg is at a 90° angle to the wall. Gently press down on your right knee with your right hand to intensify it.

What to look out for: Avoid leaning your raised knee and body toward the side being stretched, as this diminishes the effect of the stretch. Instead, try to keep your body as straight as possible while pulling the knee of the other leg in as close to the chest as possible.

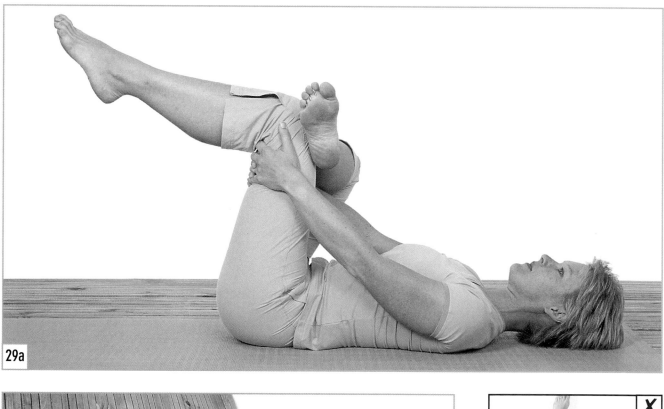

29a

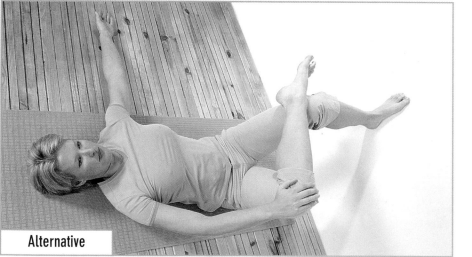

Alternative

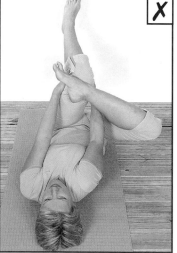

29b. Seated rotation

Type of Stretch: compound

Main Muscles: those that outwardly rotate the hip (namely the gluteals, piriformis, gemellus superior and inferior, obturator externus and internus, quadratus femoris), as well as quadratus lumborum, obliques, erector spinae and latissimus dorsi

Stretch: If your hips are tight and you find it difficult to keep your back straight in this position, sit on a folded towel or firm cushion (placed underneath both buttocks). Sit with your left leg bent, foot on the ground next to your right knee, and your right leg extended in front of you. Cross the left foot over the right knee so that it is still flat on the ground, but next to the outside of your right knee. Now bend your right leg so that your right foot is tucked up against the left buttock. With your right arm, take hold of your left knee and hug it close to your chest while you turn your torso toward the left hand side. Place your left hand on the floor for support and try to lengthen your spine. Repeat on the other side.

What to look out for: Avoid rounding the back, as this will diminish the stretch. Attempt to keep both buttocks evenly on the floor.

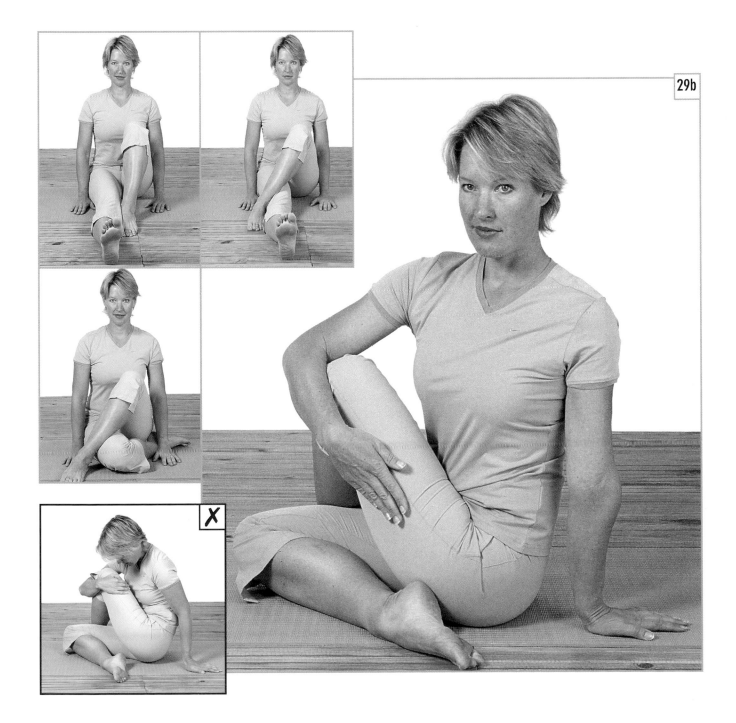

29b

X

30a. Cross-legged lean forward

Type of Stretch: compound

Main Muscles: the muscles that outwardly rotate the hip (particularly gluteus maximus)

Stretch: Sit cross-legged with your right leg in front of your left. As with the butterfly stretch, ensure that you are sitting forward on your sitting bones (*see p43 and glossary*) with your pelvis in neutral alignment, and that you are not sitting back on the flesh of your buttocks. Pull the flesh out from under your sitting bones if necessary. If your hips are tight, sit on a firm cushion or folded towel to raise them slightly. Keeping your back as straight as possible, place your hands on the floor in front of you and slowly slide them forward so that your chest moves closer and closer to the floor. You will feel this stretch in the hips.

What to look out for: As with the butterfly stretch, there is a natural tendency to want to round the back. Keeping neutral alignment of the spine will intensify the stretch and make it far more effective. Keep your shoulders depressed and make sure both buttocks rest evenly on the floor.

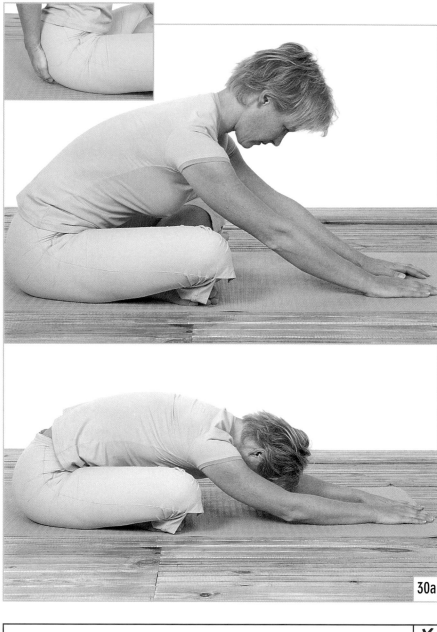

30a

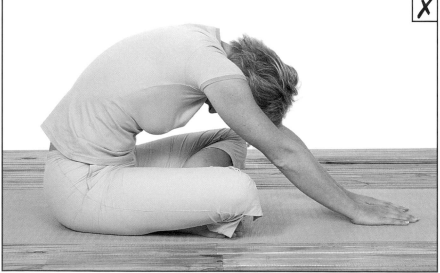

X

30b. Foot-on-knee

If you are very tight in the hips, or have a knee condition or injury, you may find this stretch uncomfortable. If this is the case, rather do the previous stretch (30a), since it targets the same areas.

Type of Stretch: compound

Main Muscles: the muscles that outwardly rotate the hip (namely the gluteals, piriformis, gemellus superior and inferior, obturator externus and internus, quadratus femoris)

Stretch: Sit cross-legged with your right leg in front. Ensure that you are sitting forward on your sitting bones (*see p43 and glossary*) with your pelvis in neutral alignment, and not on the flesh of your buttocks.

If your hips are tight, sit on a firm cushion or folded towel to raise them slightly. Place your right foot on your left knee, with the foot flexed (i.e. with the toes pulled back toward the shin). Shift your left foot forward slightly until both shins are parallel to one another and you feel the stretch in the outer hip and buttock of the right side. Place your hands behind your back and try to keep your weight evenly on both buttocks. Repeat on the other side.

What to look out for: As with the above stretch, there is a tendency to want to round the back. Keeping neutral alignment of the spine will intensify the stretch and make it far more effective.

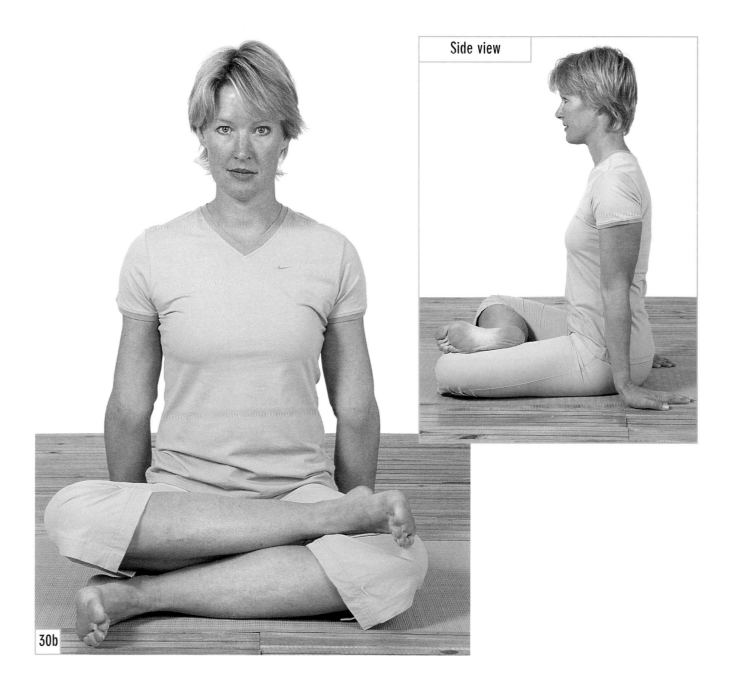

Side view

30b

31. Hip flexor stretch

Type of Stretch: compound

Main Muscles: iliopsoas and quadriceps

Stretch: With your right side next to a wall, kneel on your left knee and put your right foot flat on the ground about 75cm (30in) to one metre (40in) in front of you. If you find this uncomfortable, kneel on a towel or blanket. Place your right hand on the wall for balance and push your hips forward toward your front foot. When you start to feel a stretch at the front of your left hip, shift your right foot, so that your right ankle is directly underneath your right knee, in order to avoid unnecessary strain over the kneecap. Repeat on the other side.

What to look out for: Avoid leaning backward and thus compressing the lumbar spine; rather, lean forward slightly and lengthen the back as much as possible.

31

UPPER LEG

Mobilization

LEG SWING (*see p67*)

KNEE BEND

Gently bend your knees and lower yourself into a half sitting position. Straighten your legs again. Repeat five to eight times.

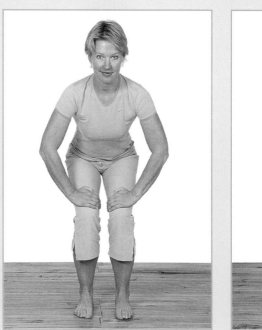
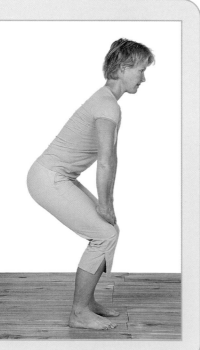

32a. Seated hamstring stretch

If you are excessively tight in your hamstrings, and are physically unable to sit with your legs straight ahead of you, you can do the lying hamstring stretch (32b) instead.

Type of Stretch: compound

Main Muscles: hamstrings and gastrocnemius

Stretch: Sit on the floor with your legs straight ahead of you. If your hamstrings feel tight, sit on a firm cushion or a folded towel. Ensure that you are sitting forward on your sitting bones (*see p43 and glossary*) with your pelvis in neutral alignment, and that you are not sitting back on the flesh of your buttocks. If you are able, take hold of your heels with your hands and, keeping your back straight and bending forward only in the hips, slowly take the front of your chest toward your feet. If your hands can't reach your feet, increase your reach by hooking a strap or belt around your heels. Keep your feet flexed, your thighs contracted and your knees straight and facing the ceiling.

If you want to increase the calf stretch, place your hands (or the strap) around the balls of your feet, instead of around your heels. The more you bring your toes back toward your chest, the more you increase the stretch – in both the hamstrings and calves.

What to look out for: Try not to round your back and hunch your shoulders during this stretch. It can be a very intense stretch, so you should try to relax and breath easily through it.

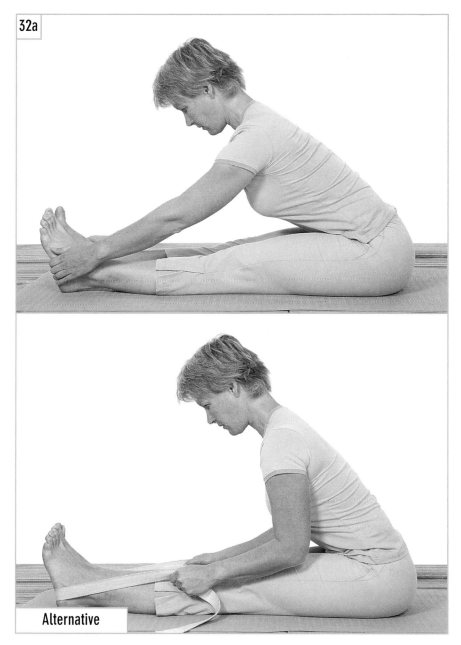

32a

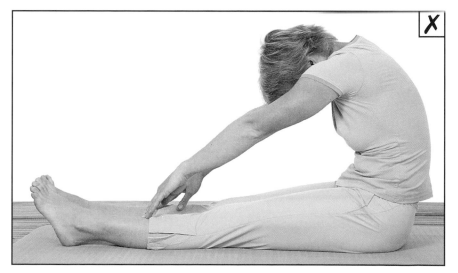

Alternative

X

32b. Lying hamstring stretch

Type of Stretch: compound

Main Muscles: hamstrings and gastrocnemius

Stretch: Lie on your back with both legs on the floor, knees straight. Bend your right leg and, if you are able, hold your foot in both hands. Slowly raise your heel up to the ceiling, straightening the knee of your raised leg until you feel a stretch behind the knee/calf/thigh. If you are unable to hold your foot,

place a strap around the heel of that same leg and hold both ends in your hands. The knee of the leg on the floor should also remain straightened, with foot flexed and toes pointing to the ceiling, and the thigh contracted.

What to look out for: Avoid bending the bottom leg; rather, use it to anchor the body, thus ensuring that the pelvis remains in neutral alignment, as opposed to rolling into a posterior tilt (*see pelvic tilt pp27 and 87*), as it is inclined to do in this position.

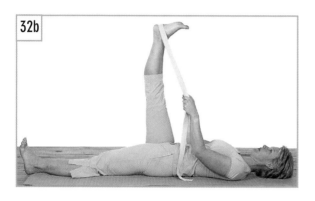

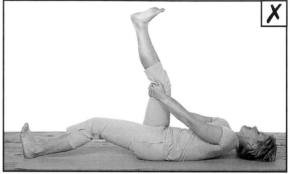

33. Downward dog stretch

Type of Stretch: compound

Main Muscles: hamstrings, gastrocnemius, soleus (if performed with bent knees), latissimus dorsi, teres major, rhomboids, mid-trapezius, triceps, posterior deltoid and pectorals

Stretch: Kneel on all fours, with your hands slightly in front of your shoulders (i.e. on a diagonal line) and your knees directly underneath your hips. Tuck your toes under so that they are flat on the floor and then raise your hips upward toward the ceiling until your knees are straight. (If your hamstrings are very tight, keep your knees bent in this stretch.) Without arching your back, push your chest toward the floor as you raise your buttocks toward the ceiling, so that your body makes a V-shape. Slowly lower your heels down onto the floor so that you feel a stretch in the calves as well as in the hamstrings, back and shoulders. Attempt to achieve a neutral spine (i.e. with a slight lumbar curvature) in order to increase the stretch in the hamstrings and calves.

What to look out for: A common error in this stretch is to over-arch the lower back, which diminishes the stretch on the back and causes unwanted compression in the lumbar region.

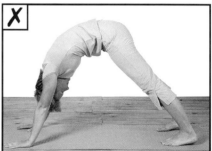

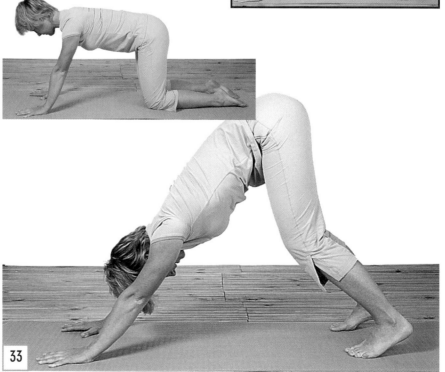

34a. Standing thigh stretch

Type of Stretch: compound

Main Muscles: quadriceps and iliopsoas

Stretch: Stand next to a wall or chair so that you can support yourself with your left hand, if necessary. Put your weight on your left leg and bend your right knee to lift your foot behind you. Take your foot in your right hand and pull it up toward your buttocks. Keep your left leg straight. Pull your navel toward your spine and ensure that your knees stay next to each other as you gently push your pubic bone forward and lengthen your spine. The stretch should be felt across either the front of the thigh or the hip of the bent leg, or possibly both. Repeat on the other side.

What to look out for: Avoid arching the lower back and always use the same hand as the leg you are stretching to hold the foot. Using either the opposite, or both hands, can cause arching of (and thus compression in) the lumbar spine.

34b. Kneeling thigh stretch (advanced)

Type of Stretch: compound

Main Muscles: quadriceps and iliopsoas

Stretch: Kneel on your left knee next to a wall so that you can put your right hand on the wall for balance. Put your right foot in front of your right hip so that it forms an angle slightly greater than 90°. The foot should be slightly in front of the knee, so that when you lean forward the knee ends up directly above the ankle, forming a 90° angle. Keeping your right hand on the wall for balance, take hold of the left foot with the left hand, and pull it toward your left buttock. Simultaneously pull your navel in toward your spine and lean forward in the right leg until you feel a stretch across either the front of the left thigh, or hip. If you are tight in both muscle groups, you may feel it in both areas. Repeat on the other side.

What to look out for: Keep the chest tilted slightly forward to ensure that the lower back is not arched excessively. For the same reason, it is also very important to keep your abdominals activated during this stretch.

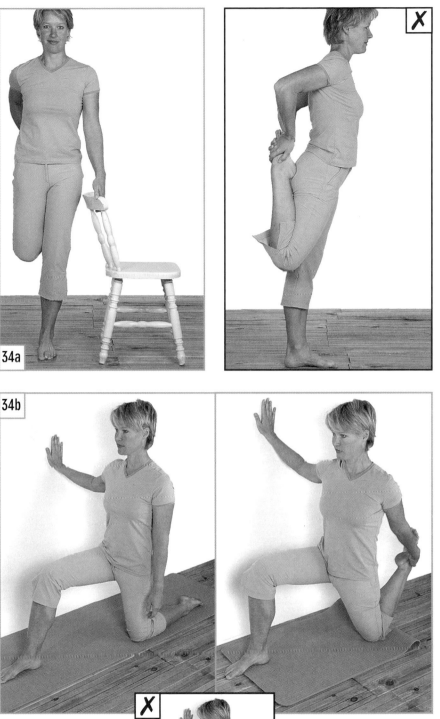

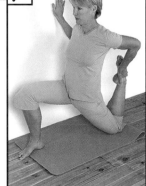

UPPER LEG

34c. Kneeling two-legged thigh stretch

As with the above stretch, if you have any knee condition or injury that makes it uncomfortable when bearing too much weight in full flexion, rather stay with the 'standing thigh stretch' (34a).

Type of Stretch: compound

Main Muscles: quadriceps and iliopsoas

Stretch: Kneel on the ground with your knees slightly apart and sit back on your heels with your hands behind your back. Gently and slowly raise your pelvis toward the ceiling. The further back you take your hands and, at the same time, the higher you lift your pelvis, the more you will feel this stretch in the targeted area. If you feel any discomfort on the inside of the knees, take them a little wider. Keep your head facing the front.

What to look out for: Avoid arching the back, rather contract the abdominal muscles while pushing up the pelvis.

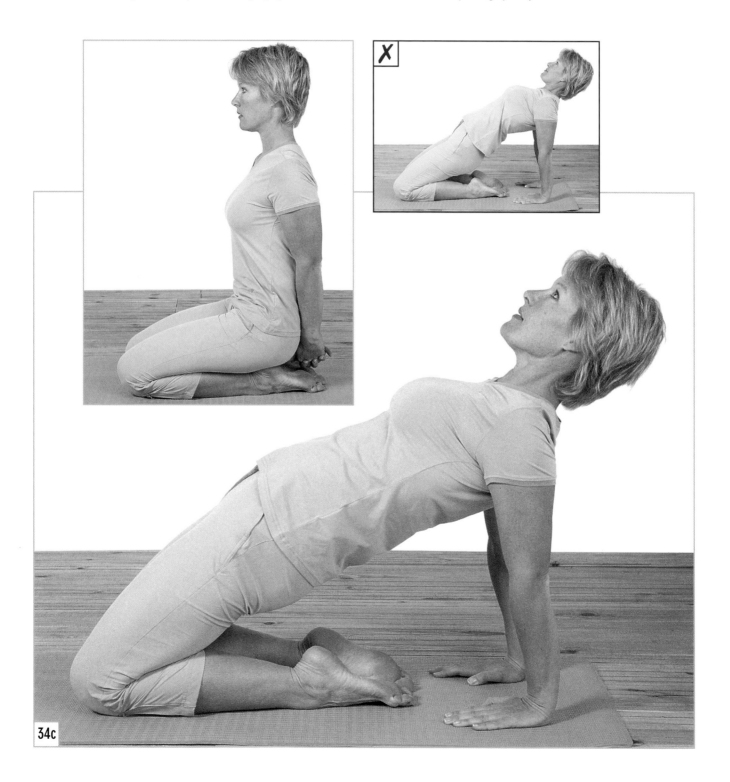

34c

35a. Seated stride

Type of Stretch: compound

Main Muscles: the leg adductors, which pull the legs together (the adductor magnus, brevis and longus of the inner thigh, as well as the pectineus, which lies in front of the pubis) and the hamstrings.

Stretch: Sit on the floor, with your legs straight and opened as wide as you comfortably can. Ensure that you are sitting forward on your sitting bones (*see p43 and glossary*) with your pelvis in neutral alignment, and that you are not sitting back on the flesh of your buttocks. If your hips are tight, sit on a firm cushion or folded towel to raise them slightly. Keeping this position and holding your calves with your hands, gently move your chest toward your feet, keeping your spine elongated. If you are unable to touch your calves without your back rounding and your pelvis rolling backward, simply keep your hands on the floor behind your buttocks, so that you can gently push the pelvis forward and straighten up the back. Ensure that your feet point upward to the ceiling at all times. The stretch should be felt in the inner thighs.

What to look out for: If you experience pain on the inside of your knee during this stretch, it may be that your legs are too wide apart.

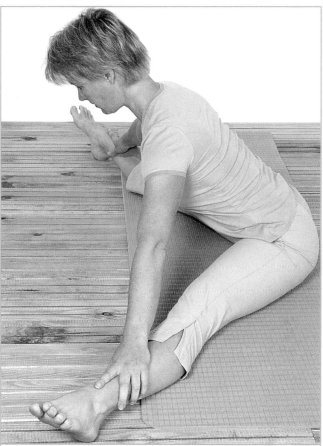

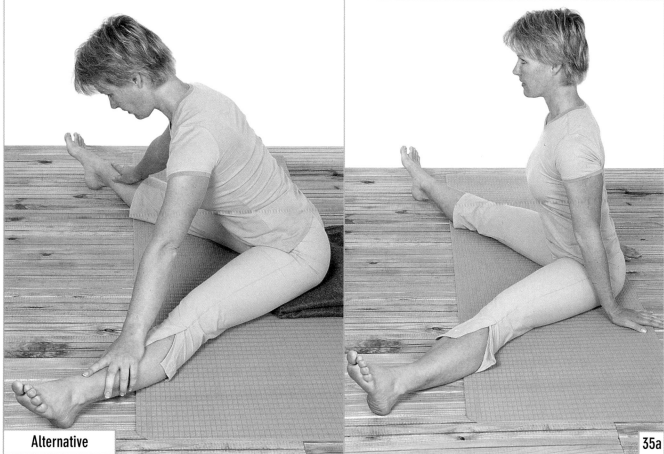

Alternative

35a

35b. Lying stride

Type of Stretch: compound

Main Muscles: the leg adductors, which pull the legs together (namely the adductor magnus, brevis and longus of the inner thigh, as well as the pectineus, which lies in front of the pubis) and, to a lesser extent, the hamstrings

Stretch: Lie on your back and lift your legs until your feet are directly above your hips. If your hamstrings are tight, you may need to loop a strap around your heels, the ends held in your hands, to keep your legs in the optimal position. Slowly open your legs as wide as you are able, keeping your feet in line with your hips (i.e. not falling forward of or behind them). If you are not using a strap, place your hands around the inside of your knees and gently apply outward pressure to your legs. When you have completed the stretch, bring your legs together before lowering them to the floor.

What to look out for: Ensure that your legs do not fall toward the floor during this stretch, since this may result in an arching of the lower back due to the discrepancy between abdominal strength and the weight of the legs.

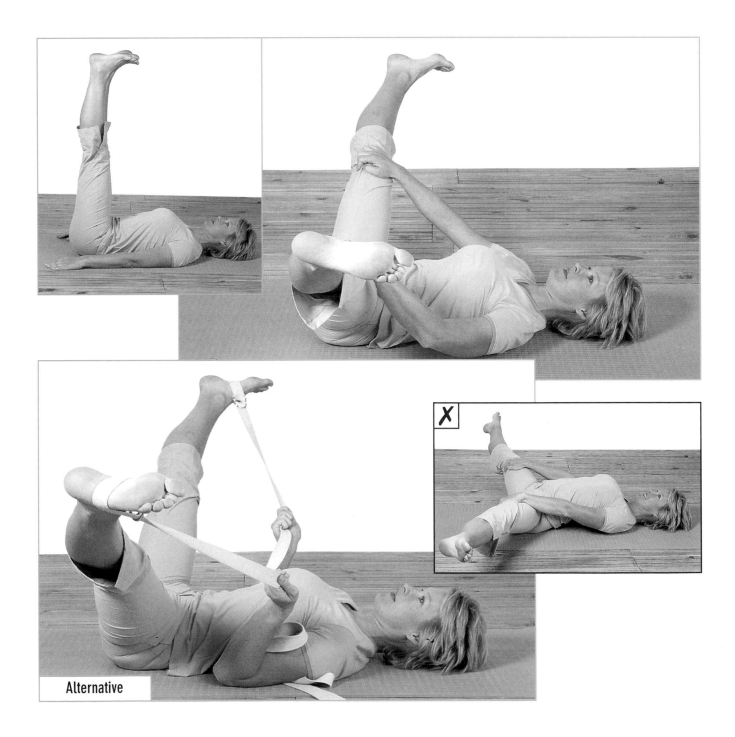

Alternative

36. ITB stretch

Although the ITB is not a muscle (it is in fact a tendon), it does sometimes tighten up with certain activities (many runners experience ITB pain or tightness) and is therefore important to stretch. This band runs from the buttocks to just below the knee joint, on the outside of the leg. Tightness in this tendon will present itself as pain or discomfort in this area.

Type of Stretch: compound

Main Muscles: iliotibial band (ITB), gluteus medius and minimus and, to a lesser degree, the tensor fasciae latae.

Stretch: Lie on your left side on the edge of a bench or table, with your back to the edge, your right arm extended above your head. Your left leg should be bent slightly so that your knee is on the bench in front of you. Keep your balance by placing your left arm on the bench or table in front of you or wrapped around your waist. With your left knee facing directly forward, take the right leg back slightly and slowly allow it to drop over the edge behind you toward the floor. If you are tight in this area, you will feel a stretch into the side and top of the left leg. Repeat on the other side.

What to look out for: Do not allow your top hip or shoulder to roll backward when you take the top leg behind and below the bottom one, as this will diminish the stretch.

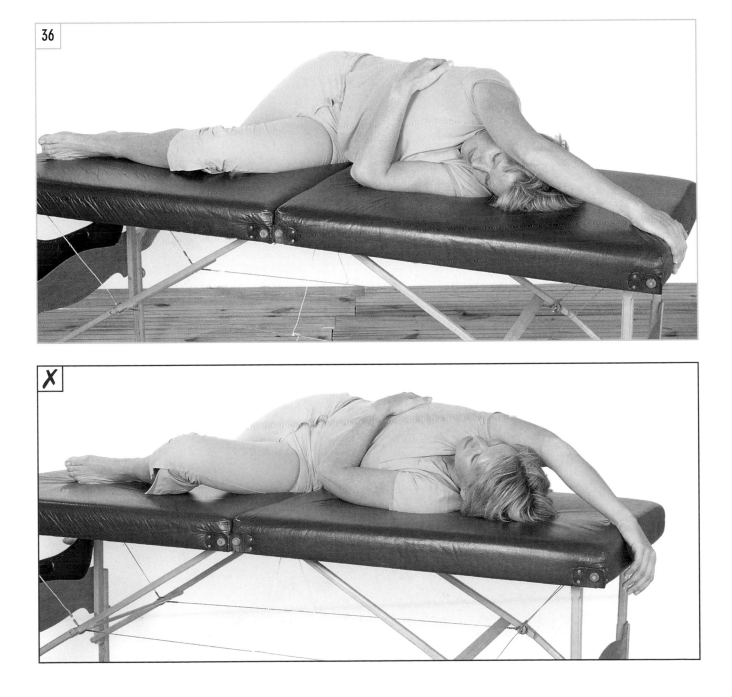

LOWER LEG AND ANKLE

Mobilization

KNEE BEND (*see p74*)

ANKLE ROLL

Slowly roll your right foot in a circle, moving first one way and then the other. Repeat five to eight times each way. Repeat on the left leg.

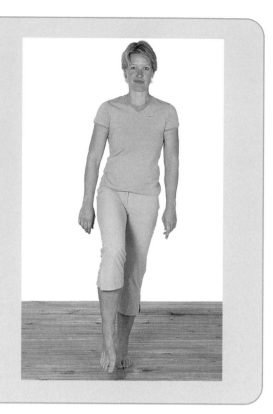

37a. Heel dip

Type of Stretch: isolation

Main Muscle: gastrocnemius

Stretch: Stand with your feet together on a step, supporting yourself with one hand on a wall or doorpost. Slide the left foot back until the heel is over the edge. Bend the right knee slightly and slowly lower the left heel until you feel a stretch in your calf. Repeat on the other side.

What to look out for: Avoid putting too much weight onto the hanging heel; you should lower yourself into the stretch gently.

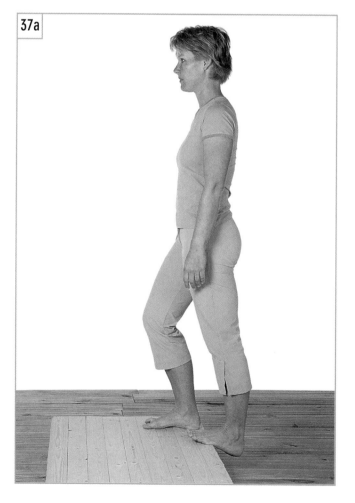

37b. Double heel dip

Type of Stretch: isolation

Main Muscle: gastrocnemius

Stretch: Stack a few books against a wall. Place one end of a large book (or a flat board) on the stack, with the end nearest you on the floor so that the slope faces you. Stand facing the wall and, while supporting yourself with your palms against the wall, place your feet on the slope (the further up the slope you place your feet, the more you will feel the stretch in your calves). Keep your feet parallel, although they can be slightly open, if this feels more comfortable. Keep your hands on the wall for support and maintain an upright position in the torso while you gently ease into this stretch.

What to look out for: Avoid allowing your buttocks to stick out behind you. If the stretch feels too intense, rather keep more of your feet on the floor than on the slope, until your calves start to loosen up.

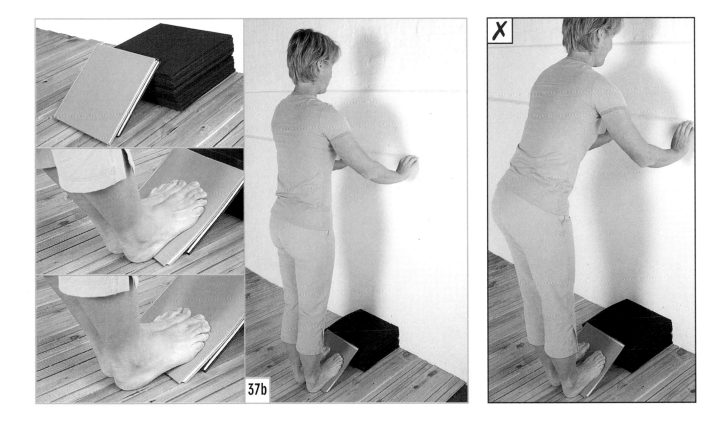

38. Heel-down knee bend

Type of Stretch: isolation

Main Muscle: soleus

Stretch: Stand with your feet together, slide one foot about 30cm (12in) behind the other, keeping the feet parallel. Keeping your weight on your back foot, bend both knees until you feel a stretch in the calf of your back leg. Repeat on the other side.

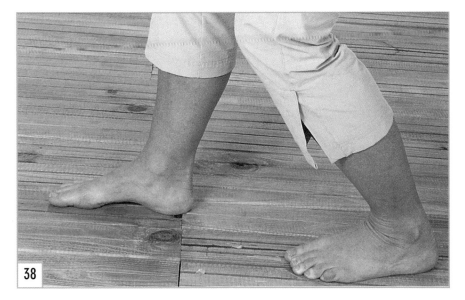

39. Top-of-toe stretch

Type of Stretch: compound

Main Muscles: tibialis anterior, peroneus tertius, extensor digitorum longus, extensor hallucis longus

Stretch: Sit in a chair with your knees and feet slightly apart. Tuck your toes under so that they are against the floor (soles of the feet are facing one another) and gently push down.

Most of your weight should be on the four smaller toes, so that the stretch is felt into the tops of those toes and across the sides of your foot and into your shin. Now draw the knees and ankles together, keeping all the toes on the floor, only this time, place more weight on your big toes. Again, push down gently, feeling the stretch across the front of your foot and into your shin.

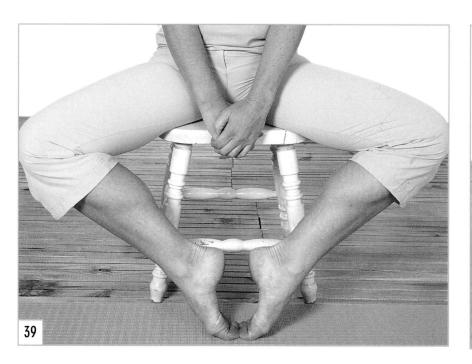

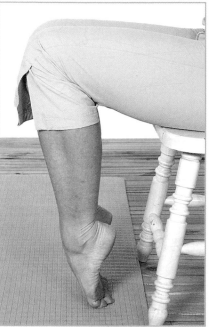

40. Bottom-of-toe stretch

Type of Stretch: compound

Main Muscles: flexor digitorum longus, flexor hallucis longus

Stretch: With the legs slightly wider than hip distance apart, stand on the left leg and place the ball of the right foot on the floor. Raise the ankle of the right foot as high as you can, and push gently forward into the toes. This stretch will be felt underneath the toes. Repeat on the other side.

What to look out for: Avoid allowing the foot to drop outward, because this will detract from the stretch.

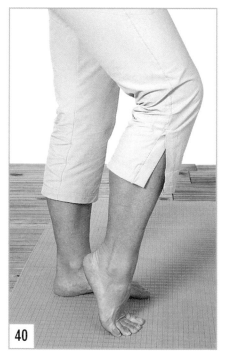

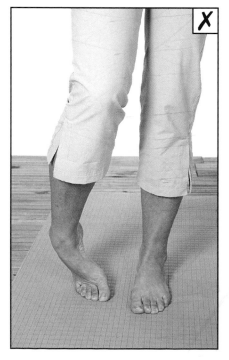

41. Outer ankle stretch

Type of Stretch: compound

Main Muscles: peroneus longus, brevis and tertius, extensor digitorum longus

Stretch: With the legs hip distance apart, stand on the left leg and roll the ankle of the right leg outward until you feel a stretch on the outside of this area. Repeat on the other side.

What to look out for: Avoid placing too much weight on the ankle joint. Instead, control the stretch by keeping most of your weight on the supporting leg.

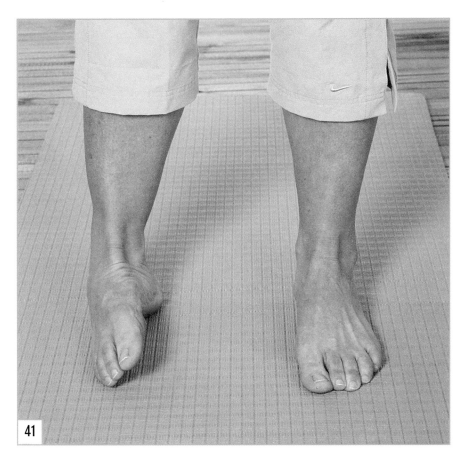

42. Inner ankle stretch

Type of Stretch: compound

Main Muscles: tibialis anterior and posterior, flexor digitorum longus, flexor hallucis longus.

Stretch: With the legs hip distance apart, stand on the left leg and roll the ankle of the right leg inward until you feel a stretch on the inside of this area. Repeat on the other side.

What to look out for: As with the outer ankle stretch, avoid placing too much weight on the ankle joint. Instead, control the stretch by keeping most of your weight on your supporting leg.

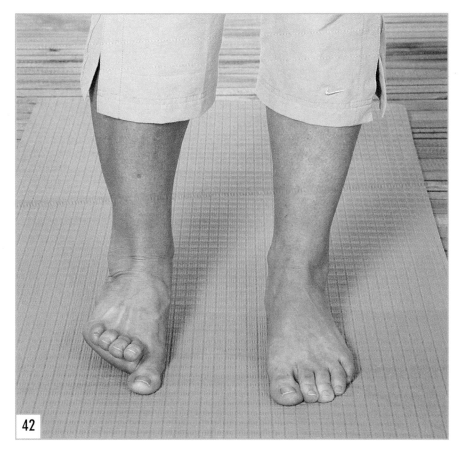

Stretching for a Healthier Lifestyle

(4)

Changing your lifestyle can be a challenging experience. For this change to be sustainable it is important to ensure that your newly adopted habits are realistic, enjoyable and have a purpose. If you can relate to any of the reasons below for including regular stretching in your life, you can be sure that this change will be a positive experience. Writing down your goals will help to keep you motivated. Enlist the help of your partner, family or work colleagues so that you have an effective emotional support base.

STRETCHING FOR BETTER POSTURE AND A HEALTHIER BACK

Many people experience pain somewhere along the spine; most frequently in the lower back (lumbar spine). There could be a number of reasons for this:

- incorrect posture resulting in a muscular imbalance (muscles that are shortened tend to be stronger than their antagonist muscles)
- tight back extensor muscles (erector spinae) causing vertebral disc compression
- weak abdominal muscles, which fail to support the lower back
- lack of mobility – an inability to bend either sideways, forward or backward
- an abnormality or injury in the lumbar spine or greater spine

The self-assessment in Chapter 2, under the heading Trunk, can help you establish whether your posture puts your pelvis in an anterior or posterior tilt (*see diagram 1*).

If you stand with an anterior pelvic tilt, your lumbar spine is probably arched. The pelvis tilts forward, decreasing the angle between the pelvis and the thigh. This narrower angle results in the shortening of the hip flexor muscles (iliopsoas). Usually, the opposing muscle groups (in this case the hamstrings and buttocks) and the abdominals will become elongated and weak. Stretching the

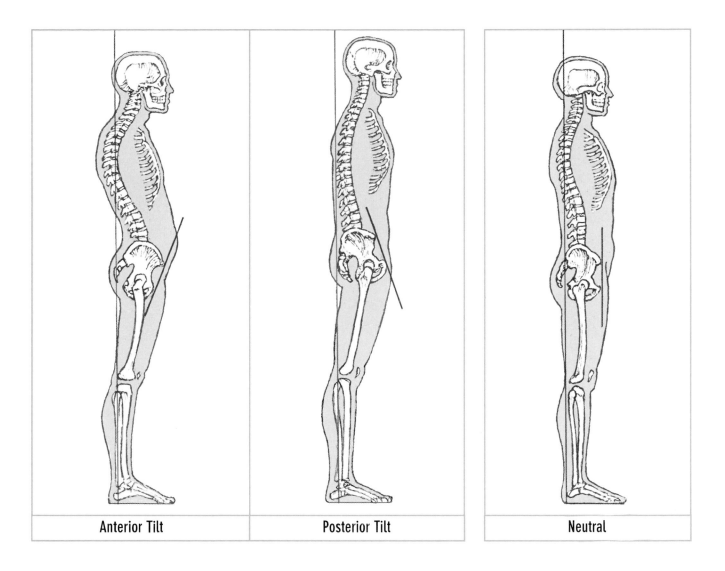

| Anterior Tilt | Posterior Tilt | Neutral |

Diagram 1   Diagram 2

short muscles regularly will improve your posture over time and the lengthened muscles, in turn, will start to strengthen as your posture changes. You can speed up the recovery by doing strengthening exercises for the lengthened muscles while you stretch the tightened ones.

If you stand with a posterior pelvic tilt, the top of the hipbone is held further back, flattening the natural curve in the lower back. The abdominals tend to be contracted. This pelvic position narrows the angle between the back of the leg and the hip, putting the hamstrings into a shortened position. The lengthened muscle groups in this case would be the back extensors, hip flexors and quadriceps, which would all be loosened and thus in need of strengthening. Simple stretches can elongate the tight muscles, allowing a natural tightening of the opposing muscles, thus re-establishing the body's natural muscular balance.

The ideal pelvic position is when the tops of the hipbones lie neither significantly in front of nor behind the pubic bone. This does not mean,

however, that the spine is flat; the natural design of our spine has a slight lumbar and thoracic curvature (*see diagram 2*). Together, these curves act as a shock absorber. If the back were ramrod straight, there would be no spring or flexibility to absorb even the impact of each footfall, let alone in the event of falling on your backside.

The second test in the self-assessment section, still under the heading Trunk, deals with spine flexibility. Ideally, you should be flexible in all three areas of the spine – the cervical spine (neck and upper back), the thoracic spine (mid back) and the lumbar spine (lower back).

Tightness in the cervical spine can lead to compression of the vertebral discs in the neck, sometimes causing headaches or neck pain. People in sedentary occupations, or who sit in front of a computer most of the day, often experience tightness in this area. Regardless of how hard you try to remain aware of your posture, this focus diminishes as you get caught up in the stress of the day. Many people have a tendency to slouch when not consciously thinking about their posture. Slouching strains the neck muscles, which have to hold the weight of the head as the chin juts forward, the head tilts upward, the shoulders roll inward and the spine becomes rounded. This muscle strain takes the form of a contraction – the muscle is pulled into a shortened position – until you either change your posture, or you stretch the muscle out.

When the thoracic spine is immobile, it can result in a hunchback effect. This is often exacerbated by tightness in the chest, which closes the front of the body, making it hard to sit or stand upright and breathe effectively.

Apart from pelvic position, tightness in the lumbar spine can also reduce spinal mobility. A person whose extensor muscles are tight will tend to bend from the hip, instead of from the spine, when leaning forward. While this is not a problem in the short term, it does mean that the lumbar spine is flexed less often, and will thus become increasingly immobile.

Good posture can help improve your breathing and general movement, and can also decrease the risk of injury because of improved nimbleness and balance. Try and create ways to remind yourself to do some simple, basic stretches throughout your day, targeting those areas you know to be tight. On page 119 there are some basic office stretches, which can be done anywhere. It is important to become aware of your posture as often as possible and to counter the damaging effects of long periods of inactivity by standing or moving frequently.

When lifting heavy objects, keep your knees bent and your abdominals contracted. This protects your lower back from bearing the compounded strain of gravity against a load.

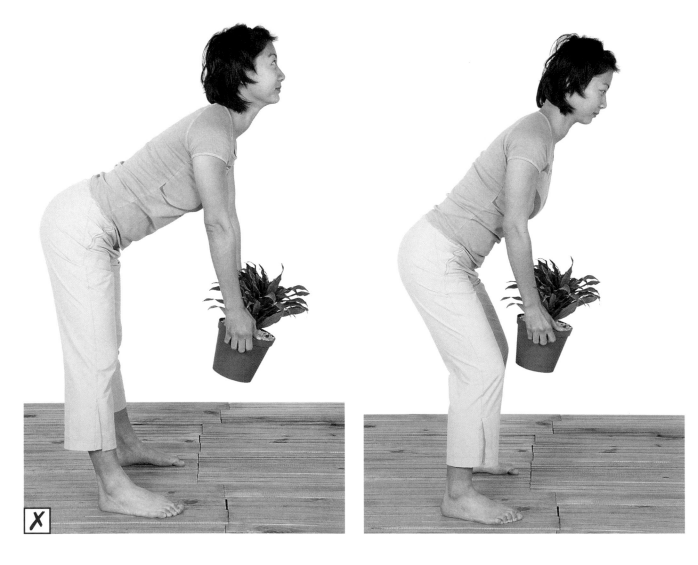

Lifting incorrectly with straight knees   Lifting correctly with bent knees

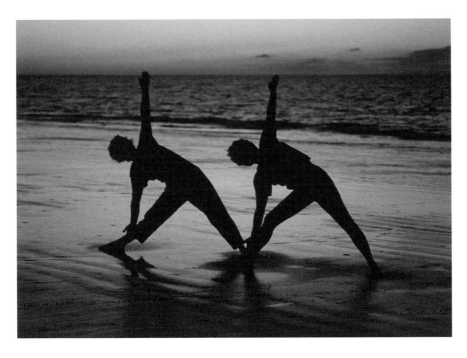

Stretching is a great way to bring some stillness to your physical body, your mind and soul.

STRETCHING TO ALLEVIATE STRESS

In the days of the caveman life was pretty simple. You went out hunting, taking great care not to become the hunted. If you crossed the path of a hungry, man-eating animal with sharp claws and a toothy grin, you would have got a fright, possibly freezing for just a second, debating rapidly the safety offered by the tree behind you, or the river in front of you. Simultaneously, your body would undergo all sorts of physiological changes – from a racing heartbeat and increased air supply (delivering more oxygen to the working muscles) to a decrease in the sex hormones (no need for these when you're in fear of your life) and a heightening of your senses. In addition to this, the blood will thicken and as much as possible will be diverted to the working muscles (to carry the additional oxygen to the muscles). A hormone, glucagon, is released by the pancreas, which increases blood sugar. There will also be an increase in cholesterol, thyroxin (a hormone released by the thyroid that regulates metabolism), cortisone (the body's natural anti-inflammatory) and endorphins (the brain's natural opiate that reduces pain and promotes euphoria and pleasure). You may stand and fight if you're trapped (or think you stand a chance of defending yourself) or, more than likely, you would run – faster than you ever thought possible, until you were safe (or eaten).

Once secure and out of danger, you would allow yourself to relax, to breathe deeply and regularly; calming yourself until you were ready to move on again. Running for your life (or fighting) would have had the positive effect of using up the increased blood supply with its cargo of hormones and energy.

These days, however, things are very different. Our stress comes in the form of a demanding boss or an overdue deadline. While the thought of running away might have its appeal, it is probably not an appropriate action given the long-term career implications. The consequences of activating your stress response (the fight-or-flight response) without the opportunity for your body to use up the energy and hormones made available by it can be accumulative and, over time, quite devastating.

Our stressors can also arrive in a more camouflaged manner, such as being frustrated by a simple task which seems beyond you; feeling as though you are losing control over your workload; or not getting the promotion for which you were in line. Often these more insidious stressors can leave your body feeling wound up; your muscles tense or in spasm.

Effective ways of coping with stress are: pounding away on a treadmill, breathing deeply, meditating, talking about your feelings and frustrations, or just having fun.

The benefit of stretching in dealing with negative stress, is that it entails physically lengthening tense or tight muscles, ultimately causing a relaxation response.

A stretch class is usually conducted in a calming manner in a quiet environment, often with relaxing and soothing music. These classes often include breathing techniques and meditation. Breathing correctly can help ease muscular tension and ensure that optimal amounts of oxygen are delivered where needed. Meditation can help regulate your heartbeat and decrease your blood pressure.

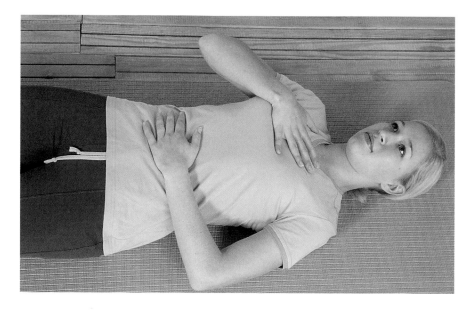

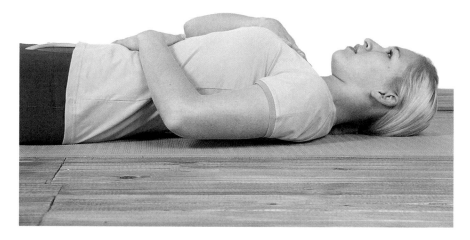

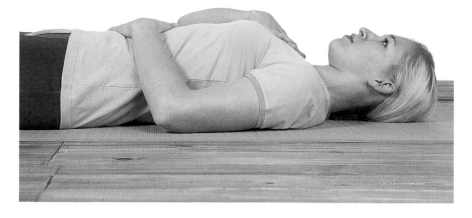

BREATHING

When people are tense they tend to take short, shallow breaths. You may have noticed that after doing something relaxing, such as having a massage, your breathing is easier and deeper. Another excellent way to ensure depth to your breathing is to exercise – you may have experienced the out-of-breath feeling that comes with exerting yourself and the feeling of wellbeing that comes with it.

Become aware of how you breathe when you are tense:

- Do your shoulders tense up, or do you lift them as you breathe in?
- Do you take short, shallow breaths?
- Do your shoulders and upper chest move with your breathing, or your abdomen?

Practice the breathing exercise described below daily, even if only for five minutes each time, and attempt to increase your awareness of your breathing throughout the day if you are tense and prone to shallow breathing. This is an excellent technique for the alleviation of general stress and to induce calmness, such as when you find yourself in the middle of an argument or when you are feeling frustrated. You can also use it to dispel specific stress or tension, by visualizing, for example, the tightness in your back or neck easing with every exhalation.

Lie on your back with your legs and arms flat on the floor in a relaxed position, with your eyes and mouth loosely closed. Place one hand on your navel and another on your chest. Take a deep breath in through your nose, filling up your abdomen so that it expands (you should be able to feel the hand over your navel rise). Now move your breath from the stomach into your chest, feeling your ribs expanding as you go (the hand over your chest should rise). Your shoulders may lift slightly, but avoid tensing them or your neck during this exercise.

Reverse the movement as you exhale, so that the breath leaves your chest first and then your abdomen, causing your navel to sink.

Count slowly so that your inhalation and exhalation are of equal duration. Aim to complete a full cycle in about 10 to 15 seconds.

MEDITATION

Although there are many different techniques, the goal of meditation is always the same – to bring stillness to the mind and consciousness to thought. Meditation provides a quiet space for reflection and calmness. Without specifically making the time to practise this technique, and especially given our rushed and jam-packed lives, we tend to move further and further away from our ability to connect with ourselves; to understand and know who we truly are. It is a tool for self-development; a road to greater awareness.

The following technique is simple and can be done anywhere, anytime.

Sit in a place where you are comfortable and warm, in a position that allows you to be still with a relaxed body and neutral spine. Most people seem to be comfortable in the cross-legged position, but if you have tight hips, sit up on a cushion so that your hips are elevated and your pelvis is able to find a neutral position easily enough (that is, not rolled forward or backward).

You can concentrate on your own breathing, or an object. If you are using an object, place it where you can see it without having to turn your head. Glance at it from time to time through your meditation, attempting to keep the image in your mind's eye after you have closed your eyes.

If you are concentrating on your breathing, try and ensure that it is quiet and regular. You might want to mentally repeat a word or phrase, using the same rhythm as your breathing in order to help with regularity and focus.

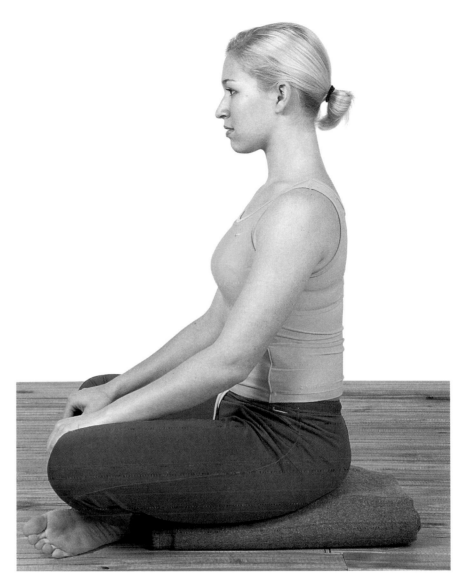

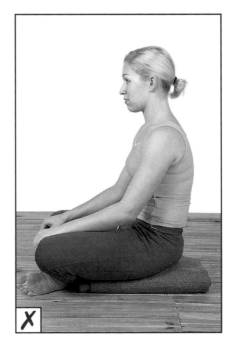

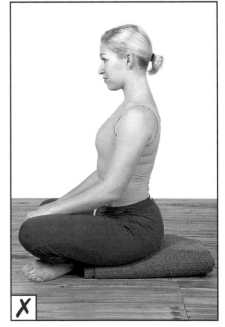

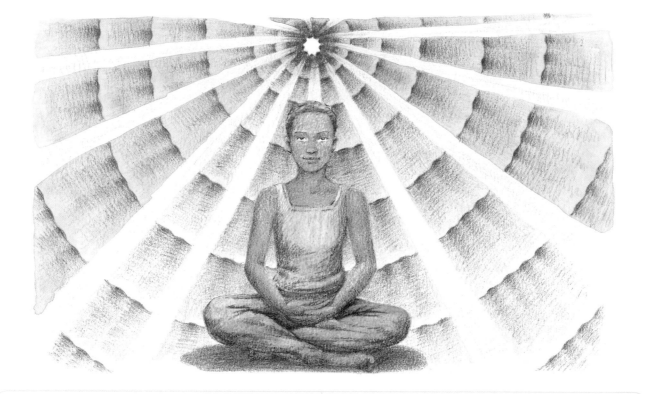

Try a stilling and centring technique before your meditation. Merwede van der Merwe, in her book *Meditation: a path to consciousness*, suggests the following preparation exercise for stilling the mind and centring awareness:

1. Sit in a comfortable position with a straight spine, hands on your lap, relaxed, palms upward. Relax your body. Close your eyes. Be aware of your breathing.

2. Focus your awareness inward. Let go of the outside world. Experience yourself in the moment.

3. Mentally release the weight of your body. Imagine that your body is melting into the ground. Just let go.

4. Scan your body, feeling the softness in each part: your feet and legs, buttocks, hips, abdomen, chest, shoulders, arms and hands. Feel that your head is balanced. Relax your jaw; soften your whole face.

5. Extend your spine upward toward the crown of your head. Allow your chest to open at the same time.

6. Be fully aware of your whole body. Notice any sensations. Accept the way your body is feeling. Remain focused on your body for two to three minutes.

7. Now focus your attention on your breathing. Feel the inhalations and the exhalations. Notice the rhythm of expansion and contraction. Do not interfere with your breathing; just watch it for two to three minutes.

8. Now open your awareness fully to the environment. Notice any aromas, feel the atmosphere around you. Listen to all the sounds, near and far. Pay attention to all external stimuli for two to three minutes.

9. Bring your awareness back to your body. Focus on your breathing. Feel the gentle movement of air in your chest and in your nostrils. Feel the rhythm.

10. Expand your awareness again to include your whole body. Feel the quietness and softness. Notice how the breath is moving in your body.

11. Pay attention to your spine, making sure that it is erect. Take a full breath and release it slowly.

12. Start the concentration technique of your choice.

Just five minutes of meditation a day will benefit you, although more will be better. Instructors often use simple meditation techniques in their yoga or stretch classes. If you practise alone, try to include some meditation, perhaps in the last five or 10 minutes of your session, so that it becomes a habit, at least every time you stretch.

You could even swap between the two techniques. Try not to respond to any distractions and, should you lose the image for a while and find that your mind starts to become busy, gently come back to it again, bearing in mind that the aim is not to have a blank mind, but rather one that is still and calm.

STRETCHING AS A FORM OF EXERCISE

Many people are not sure what type of exercise will benefit them most, especially when the time they can set aside for it is limited and they would like to make the most of what time they have available. While it would be ideal to include all three components of fitness (cardiovascular, strength and flexibility), this is not always realistic. Rather, it is essential that you opt for a form of exercise that you find enjoyable and that suits your lifestyle. Otherwise, your initial motivation and commitment will soon wane.

Remember that any activity counts – including gardening, walking your dog, or housework. Daily movement promotes good health and keeps your metabolism activated.

Most of your movements throughout the day require your muscles to contract. For that reason stretching these same muscles each day will help ensure muscular balance and efficiency. Ask yourself the following:

■ is there stiffness in any area of your body?
■ do you stand more than you sit during any given day?
■ do you enjoy activities that make you work hard, but also elongate your muscles?
■ do you enjoy quiet, calming, physical activities as opposed to beat-driven, loud and 'busy' physical activities?

If you answered 'yes' to one or more of these, chances are you would do very well on a stretching programme. The more positive answers, the more convinced you should feel about your need for such a programme.

Establish which stretches will balance the way in which your muscles are developed by your regular activities. Include these in your programme to ensure a balanced and supple body.

In order too improve your health, you should try to accumulate at least 30 minutes of physical activity at a moderate intensity each day. (Moderate exertion should leave you feeling slightly out of breath, but still able to hold a conversation.) This can be achieved by means of stretching, particularly if you are very stiff and unused to moving your muscles and joints through their full range of movement. If your goal is to improve your fitness level, you will need to commit a little more energy to your chosen exercise programme. This can also be achieved through flexibility training, but it will require a very specific type of programme.

The principle of overload states that the body needs to be stimulated beyond its current ability for a response (increased strength or fitness) to be elicited. In this case the stretch is the overload stimulus.

The principle of progression states that as your body adapts to the increased stimulus with increased strength and fitness, you'll have to increase the stimulus to see continued improvement (increase the weights or resistance for increased strength, or the distance, speed or duration for increased aerobic fitness). Your programme must be continually adapted so that it continues to challenge your body. For flexibility, this would involve adding more complex stretches.

The principle of specificity refers to the type of exercise chosen. If your aim is to be able to do the splits, running will not help you achieve this goal. Similarly, if your aim is to make it through a marathon, stretching

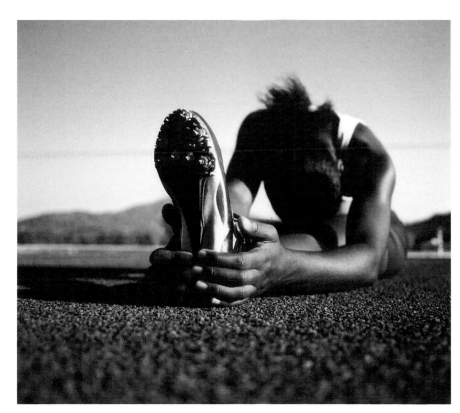

will not improve your running fitness – nor will running improve your power-lifting performance or vice versa.

The principle of reversibility states that if the challenge (as in the form of stretching) provided to the body is no longer apparent, the adaptation made by the body may be lost. The longer you've been stretching (providing the challenge) the longer it will take for the results of adaptation to wane.

Finally, the principle of FITT (frequency, intensity, type and time) provides a framework for developing a programme of comfortable exercise sessions, that will challenge you and leave you feeling refreshed, not as if you have been run over.

Frequency

This is the number of times you exercise in a week. Anything less than twice a week is not likely to give you remarkable results. On the other hand, working the same muscles every day of the week can lead to over-training injuries. Three to five times per week will give your muscles time to adapt, but without allowing the results to wane.

Intensity

This refers to how hard you work in a session. You can gauge the intensity of your workout with the Borg scale of perceived exertion:

0	Feeling nothing at all
1	Effort feels very weak
2	Effort is weak
3	Effort is moderate
4	Effort is somewhat strong
5	Effort is strong
6	/
7	Effort is very strong
9	/
10	Effort is very, very strong

For a really high intensity workout you should aim for the 7–10 range, while a moderate intensity workout will be more in the 3–6 range.

Type

This refers to the type of exercise you do. Although this book is about stretching, even within the category of flexibility training, there are different techniques you may wish to explore. Some of these include yoga, Pilates, or just a basic stretch class at the gym.

Time

This refers to the time spent exercising in one session. It has been established that 30 minutes of continuous activity at a moderate intensity is necessary to promote health, so it would not make sense to spend less time exercising than this. (Although one should not lose sight of the fact that any amount of time spent moving around during the day is better than spending all day lying on a couch.)

Applying FITT

It is, however, possible to adapt the elements of FITT to work out a programme of exercise that takes into account the time you have available and the intensity at which you exercise so that, on balance, you still get the equivalent of at least 30 minutes of exercise a day.

Let's look at some options, by throwing this FITT principle into the mix. Exercise at a lower intensity for a longer duration (intensity; time)

Or

Exercise at a high intensity for a shorter duration (intensity; time)

Or

Exercise at a lower intensity for a shorter duration, seven days a week (frequency; intensity; time)

Or

Exercise at a lower intensity for a longer duration, four times a week (frequency; intensity; time)

Or

Exercise at a higher intensity for a shorter duration, three times a week (frequency; intensity; time)

Or

Attend an advanced, high intensity 60-minute yoga class twice a week and a basic, low intensity 45-minute stretch class twice a week (frequency; intensity; type; time)

Or

Attend a moderate intensity 90-minute stretch class four times a week (frequency; intensity; type; time)

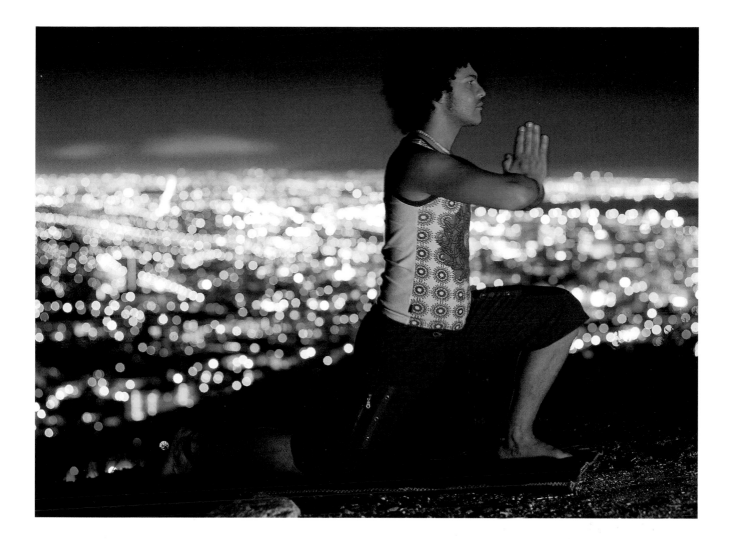

YOGA

Yoga is a well-known form of physical and spiritual practice; the essence of which is the ultimate unifying of the mind and body. Although some forms of yoga are far more physical than others, physical achievement is secondary to the benefits derived from its regular practice, irrespective of the level at which you do so. For many, the benefits of its practice are also secondary to the journey undertaken by the student — that of transcending the consciousness of the ego, and allowing one to realize the self. Yoga is, in itself, a philosophy of life, the end result of which is the creation of a vibrantly healthy body and mind.

Having said this, many people partake in yoga for its physical benefits, which include increased strength, flexibility, balance, improved circulation and a reduction in stress. It is not necessary to accept the philosophy to benefit from this aspect of the practice. Although many poses require stamina and strength, yoga is best known for improving flexibility. Because it incorporates a measure of functional resistance training (using body weight to load the muscles and develop strength), as well as flexibility training, it offers a balanced and effective workout.

Find a style of flexibility training that challenges, excites and motivates you, since the best way to ensure suppleness and postural balance is through regular and consistent practice.

Other benefits offered to women include the easing of menopausal symptoms. Many poses also ease menstrual cramps, heavy bleeding, pelvic discomfort and associated low back pain and can also be effective in calming the emotional turbulence experienced by some women during this time of their cycle. Some postures and breathing techniques also help balance the endocrine system. Women who discover these benefits and experience them personally, tend to adjust their attitudes accordingly and thus feel more empowered and energized.

An important aspect of yoga practice is breath work, which involves practising various breathing techniques. Breathing cannot be over-emphasized when practising yoga, since it facilitates all movement, and movement results in posture. Thus the endpoint of breath-work is the *asanas* (poses).

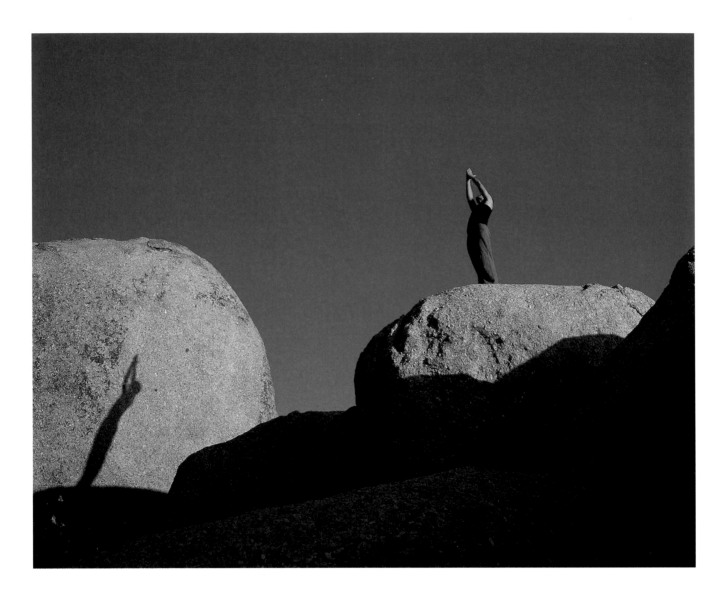

There are many different styles of yoga – some of which derive from the original forms, while others are completely independent. Listed below are some well-known yoga forms, with a description of each. Having an idea of the various philosophies involved in each style should help you decide which form appeals to you more, and which suits your personal lifestyle and your own philosophy best.

Hatha Yoga

The literal translation of *hatha* is force. As with Iyengar yoga, Hatha yoga is a very physical practice that makes use of different asanas. The intention is to strengthen the body, opening and cleansing it at the same time. The asanas are blocked together according to their movement type. For example, twists (turning the body), forward bends (working down toward the front of the body), backward bends (working toward the back of the body), inversions (parts or whole of the body upside down), standing and seated poses.

Physical activity is a vital part of anyone's life, regardless of age, fitness level or shape. The health benefits attributed to increased activity will come with dedication and commitment.

Closely resembling the eight limbs in Ashtanga yoga, Hatha yoga has eight stages or steps within its system of practice. *Yama* and *niyama* concern universal ethics and morals, as well as personal behaviour. *Asana* and *pranayama* relate to the practice of yoga postures and breath control respectively. *Pratyahara*, *dharana* and *dhyana* refer to the controlling of senses, concentration, and meditation respectively. The eighth step deals with the super-consciousness (*samadhi*), the final result of the all the ascetic's spiritual efforts and exercises. It means union, totality, absorption in, complete concentration of mind, conjunction.

Psycho-spiritually, the aim of Hatha yoga is to ensure that the body is ultimately capable of dealing with the realization of the self.

Bikram Yoga

This style of yoga involves a series of 26 demanding poses (*asanas*), which are performed in a heated environment. Since warmer muscles respond better to stretching than cold ones, the heated room facilitates deeper flexibility work. Another advantage is that the heat promotes sweating, and thus the flushing of toxins from the body. Bikram yoga is said to reduce the symptoms of many chronic diseases (such as arthritis and thyroid disorders) and teaches you to keep a focused mind and with control of breath, allowing you to work calmly and efficiently.

Ashtanga Yoga

The word *ashtanga* means eight branches or limbs, namely *yama* (abstinence), *niyama* (observances), *asana* (postures), *pranayama* (breath control), *pratyahara* (withdrawal of senses), *dharana* (concentration), *dhyana* (meditation), and *samadhi* (contemplation). The idea is that these branches support each other; the first four are seen as externally oriented limbs, which must be well rooted before the four internally oriented limbs develop. Thus, correct sequential order is important – allowing the student the eventual realization of all these attributes and life skills. More literally, this equates to the development of human consciousness on the physical, psychological and spiritual level. This style of yoga requires considerable effort to perform. Sweat, strength and stamina are aspects of this style of yoga, which is said to activate and circulate vital energy through the body, strengthening and purifying the nervous system.

Iyengar Yoga

The focus of this type of yoga is that of optimal physical alignment. It is thus a very physical exercise regime. Poses are held for a long duration so that while you are stretching one area of the body, another is being strengthened by keeping you in the position, resulting in high levels of strength, flexibility and muscle endurance. Although there is still a focus on efficient breathing, the emphasis is not as strong as it is in many other styles of yoga.

Kundalini Yoga

The word *kundalini* means coiling. The aim of this independent approach to yoga is to awaken the serpent power by means of various postures, breath control, chanting, and meditation. Georg Feuerstein, Yoga Research and Education Center, http://www.yrec.org writes that: 'In the classical literature of Hatha yoga, Kundalini is described as a coiled serpent at the base of the spine. The image of coiling, like a spring, conveys the sense of untapped potential energy. Perhaps more meaningfully, Kundalini can be described as a great reservoir of creative energy at the base of the spine.

Bhakti Yoga

The name originates from the root *bbaj*, and this style of yoga emphasizes love (of the self) and devotion. The aim of this practice is to channel one's cleansed emotional force toward the Divine. Thus, this form of yoga has a more emotional base than others; with practitioners dedicated to Bhakti, viewing the Divine as a supreme being, rather than an impersonal entity. The ultimate state is that of becoming one with God.

Jnana Yoga

The word *jnana* means knowledge or wisdom, and Jnana yoga aims to achieve self-realization by developing the wisdom required to discern reality from illusion.

Karma Yoga

This is the yoga of service to others and God. The essence of this practice is to act for the sake of action, without the need for results (in fact the results are left to God). In this way, the greater good becomes more important than personal benefit.

Mantra Yoga

Mantra yoga (relating to transformative sound) is thought to be one of the least difficult of all yoga forms, because it involves no complicated practices. Rather, its essence is one of regular and prolonged repetition of one or more powerful sounds (mantra), which apparently awaken the serpent power (*see Kundalini yoga, opposite page*).

Laya Yoga

The word *laya* comes from the root *li*, which means 'to vanish' or 'become dissolved.' It also means 'to cling' and 'to remain sticking.' Laya yoga practitioners aim to dissolve themselves spiritually through meditation, while clinging to the transcendental self. Thus meditation is a major aspect of this form.

Raja Yoga

Meaning 'royal yoga,' this is a relatively recent form. It refers to the eight steps of meditative introversion within the Hatha yoga system. According to some, the four main kinds of yoga are Mantra, Laya, Hatha, and Raja, all of which include the practices of posture, breath control and meditation.

5

Stretch Routines

If you participate in a regular activity, stretching afterward provides a good opportunity to improve your flexibility, since your muscles will be warm and your joints mobilized (*see p38*). Also, in some instances, failing to stretch certain muscles after a particular activity could result in those muscles becoming tight, causing an imbalance.

After you have fatigued your muscles or overloaded them (*see p93*) they retain a 'pump' — they appear bigger and are shortened somewhat. This is mostly due to the repetition of intense muscle activity that seldom stretches the muscle to its full extent or the joint through its full range of motion. (To do so in the heat of competition would risk injury.) The 'pumped' muscle is full of the by-products of exhaustive exercise. If the muscle is not stretched afterward, it will retain this decreased range of motion. Static stretching of the 'pumped' muscle will help it, and the related joint, to 'remember' the full range of motion.

Each activity uses different muscles in a different way and this chapter gives lists with suggested stretches to follow some of the most common recreational activities. The aim of this book is to provide information for people who exercise or participate in sport only on a recreational level. The stretches listed here by no means target every muscle used during the given activity, but only the main muscle groups.

Many of the stretches are compound (significantly stretch more than one muscle at a time), but to avoid repetition they have been listed under only one body part per programme. For example, the bent-arm wall stretch will stretch the muscles of the chest as well as those that internally rotate the shoulder joint. This stretch is however only listed under the anatomical area Chest, when in fact it is also a shoulder stretch.

The routines have been compiled to avoid repetition, while being as comprehensive and time-efficient as possible. Most of them will take about 10–15 minutes to complete if you allow about

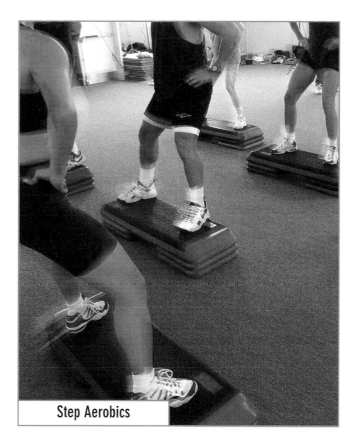

Step Aerobics

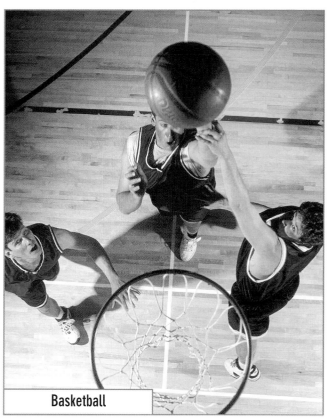

Basketball

30 seconds for each stretch. However, you are encouraged to extend your stretches if you have more time.

Note that all times are approximate depending on the stretches selected.

ACTIVITY STRETCHES

Aerobic dance and step aerobics

Calves tend to become tight and can lead to an imbalance in strength and size between the front of the shin muscle and the calf muscles, resulting in shin splints (pain along the front of the shin).

CHEST

4a. bent-arm wall stretch or

4b. doorway stretch or

4c. elbow squeeze

LOWER AND MIDDLE BACK

10. forward hanging stretch

UPPER BACK

14. snake

SHOULDERS

18. elbow up/elbow down

HIPS

29a. foot-over-knee or

29b seated rotation

30a. cross-legged lean forward or

30b. foot-on-knee

31. hip flexor stretch

UPPER LEG

32a. seated hamstring stretch or

32b. lying hamstring stretch

34a. standing thigh stretch or

34b. kneeling thigh stretch or

34c. kneeling two-legged thigh stretch

35a. seated stride or

35b. lying stride

LOWER LEG, ANKLE AND FOOT

37a. heel dip

38. heel-down knee bend

41. outer ankle stretch

42. inner ankle stretch

Duration: 12 minutes 30 seconds

Basketball

This activity requires a lot of forward flexion (crouching over) and then extension (straightening out) of the torso. Ensuring flexibility in the back and back of the legs will help to reduce tightness.

ABDOMINALS

3a. standing side stretch or

3b. seated side stretch

CHEST

4a. bent-arm wall stretch or

4b. doorway stretch or

4c. elbow squeeze

LOWER AND MIDDLE BACK

10. forward hanging stretch

11. lying torso twist

UPPER BACK

14. snake

SHOULDERS

18. elbow up/elbow down

22a. kneeling hand clasp

22b. straight-arm bridge

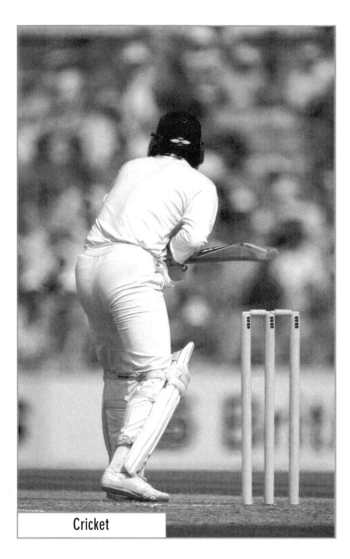

Cricket

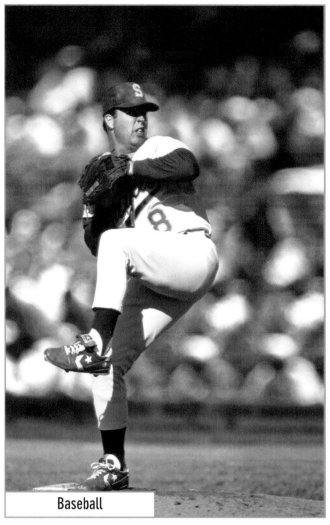

Baseball

FOREARM, WRIST AND HAND

25. kneeling wrist stretch

HIPS

28a. butterfly or

28b. squat stretch

29a. foot-over-knee or

29b. seated rotation

30a. cross-legged lean forward

31. hip flexor stretch

UPPER LEG

32a. seated hamstring stretch or

32b. lying hamstring stretch

34a. standing thigh stretch or

34b. kneeling thigh stretch or

34c. kneeling two-legged thigh stretch

35a. seated stride or

35b. lying stride

LOWER LEG AND ANKLE

37a. heel dip or

37b. double heel dip

38. heel-down knee bend

41. outer ankle stretch

42. inner ankle stretch

Duration: 15 minutes

Cricket and baseball

Depending on your position, it is likely that one side of the body is used predominantly, so add stretches and strength training exercises to ensure balance.

ABDOMINALS

3a. standing side stretch or

3b. seated side stretch or

3c. kneeling side stretch

CHEST

6. hand clasp

LOWER AND MIDDLE BACK

10. forward hanging stretch

11. lying torso twist

12a. frog stretch or

12b. standing pull-back

UPPER BACK

13a. arm-across-chest or

13b. hand-over-knee

14. snake

SHOULDERS

18. elbow up/elbow down

FOREARM, WRIST AND HAND

25. kneeling wrist stretch

26. scarecrow stretch

27. hand press

29a. foot-over-knee or

29b. seated rotation

30a. cross-legged lean forward or

30b. foot-on-knee

31. hip flexor stretch

UPPER LEG

32a. seated hamstring stretch or

32b. lying hamstring stretch

34a. standing thigh stretch or

34b. kneeling thigh stretch or

34c. kneeling two-legged thigh stretch

LOWER LEG, ANKLE AND FOOT

37b. double heel dip

38. heel-down knee bend

Duration: 14 minutes 30 seconds

Cycling/indoor cycling

Leg muscles can become very tight and, if the seat is too low, the thighs can overwork. If one already has tightness in the hamstrings, cycling can exacerbate this lack of flexibility, which can lead to tightness (and possibly pain) in the lower back.

ABDOMINALS

1a. cobra or

1b. kneeling back bend

CHEST

5. lying chest opener

7. chest press

LOWER AND MIDDLE BACK

10. forward hanging stretch

12a. frog stretch

UPPER BACK

14. snake

NECK

15. seated neck stretch

SHOULDERS

18. elbow up/elbow down

FOREARM, WRIST AND HAND

26. scarecrow stretch

27. hand press

HIPS

28a. butterfly or

28b. squat stretch

29a. foot-over-knee or

29b. seated rotation

30a. cross-legged lean forward or

30b. foot-on-knee

31. hip flexor stretch

UPPER LEG

32a. seated hamstring stretch or

32b. lying hamstring stretch

34a. standing thigh stretch or

34b. Kneeling thigh stretch or

34c. kneeling two-legged thigh stretch

35a. seated stride or

35b. lying stride

LOWER LEG, ANKLE AND FOOT

37a. heel dip or

37b. double heel dip

Duration: 13 minutes 30 seconds

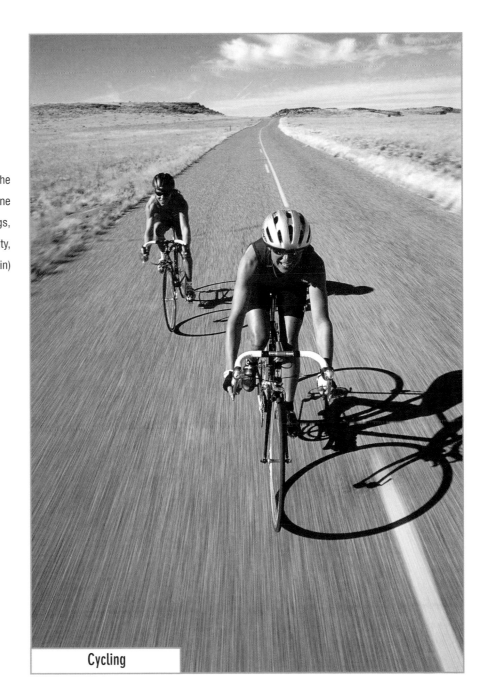

Cycling

Canoeing/rowing kayaking/paddleskiing

The back is worked significantly in this kind of exercise, so stretching the latissimus dorsi will help prevent tightness developing in the lower back. The latissimus dorsi are biggest near the lower back, so this is the area that will be affected if these muscles become over-developed. Incorrectly performed, the rowing or paddling action can also cause over-development of the neck and upper trapezius muscles. If you suspect you are using these muscles, stretch them frequently or you may find that you start to suffer from tension headaches and painful muscular knots.

ABDOMINALS

1a. cobra or

1b. kneeling back bend

3a. standing side stretch or

3b. seated stretch or

3c. kneeling side stretch

LOWER AND MIDDLE BACK

8. child pose

11. lying torso twist

12a. frog stretch or

12b. standing pull-back

UPPER BACK

13a. arm-across-chest or

13b. hand-over-knee

14. snake

SHOULDERS

18. elbow up/elbow down

19. shoulder strap stretch

20. chicken

UPPER ARM

23. straight-arm wall stretch

FOREARM, WRIST AND HAND

27. hand press

HIPS

30a. cross-legged lean forward or

30b. foot-on-knee

31. hip flexor stretch

LOWER LEG, ANKLE AND FOOT

35. top-of-toe stretch (using a foot strap)

Duration: 11 minutes 30 seconds

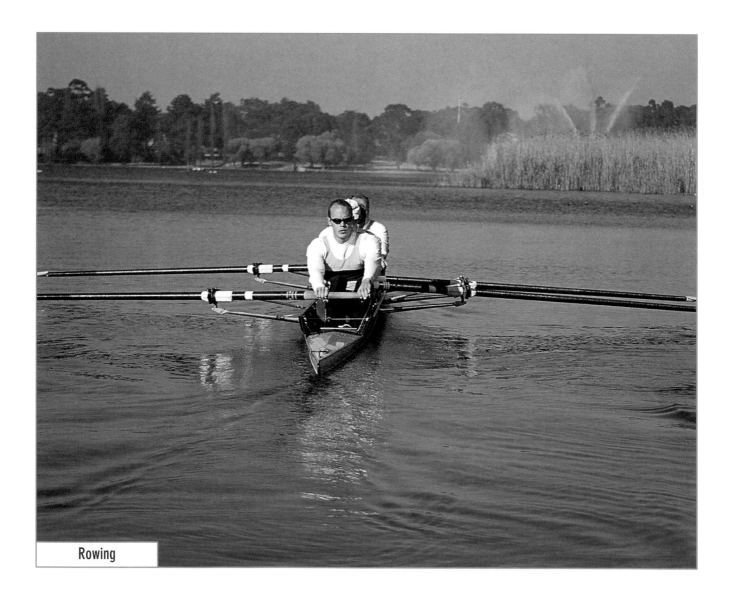

Rowing

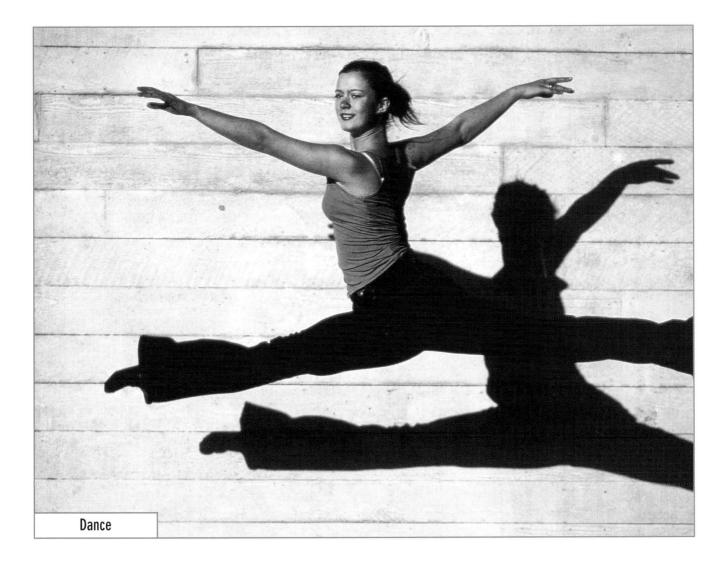

Dance

Dance

Different styles of dance will work different areas of the body. For example, ballet tends to overwork the external rotators of the hip because of the turned-out position of the feet and this could cause an imbalance in the hip. These muscles should therefore be stretched. The high-heeled shoes worn in Latin American dancing can cause back-related problems, because they affect the body's natural posture. Lower back stretches would help. Scottish and Irish folk dancing could cause lower leg imbalances since work is done on the balls of the feet. The calves should be stretched regularly.

ABDOMINALS

1a. cobra or

1b. kneeling backbend

3a. standing side stretch or

3c. kneeling side stretch

CHEST

6. hand clasp

LOWER AND MIDDLE BACK

10. forward hanging stretch

11. lying torso twist

NECK

15. seated neck stretch

HIPS

28a. butterfly or

28b. squat stretch

29a. foot-over-knee or

29b. seated rotation

30a. cross-legged lean forward or

30b. foot-on-knee

31. hip flexor stretch

UPPER LEG

32a. seated hamstring stretch or

32b. lying hamstring stretch

34a. standing thigh stretch or

34b. kneeling thigh stretch or

34c. kneeling two-legged thigh stretch

35a. seated stride or

35b. lying stride

LOWER LEG, ANKLE AND FOOT

37a. heel dip or

37b. double heel dip

38. heel-down knee bend

40. bottom-of-toe stretch

41. outer ankle stretch

42. inner ankle stretch

Duration: 15 minutes 30 seconds

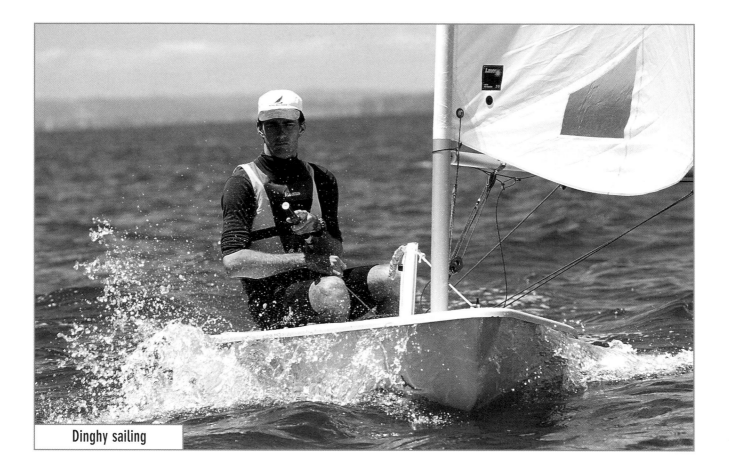

Dinghy sailing

Dinghy sailing

The crew often 'hikes out in trapeze,' (leaning over the side of the boat to counter-balance the force of the wind on the sails). This requires very strong abdominals and can work your back for you. They should stretch abdominals, latissimus dorsi and biceps.

ABDOMINALS

1a. cobra or

1b. kneeling back bend

LOWER AND MIDDLE BACK

10. forward hanging stretch

12a. frog stretch or

12b. standing pull-back

UPPER BACK

13a. arm-across-chest

13b. hand-over-knee

SHOULDERS

19. shoulder strap stretch

UPPER ARM

23. straight-arm wall stretch

FOREARM, WRIST AND HAND

25. kneeling wrist stretch

26. scarecrow stretch

27. hand press

HIPS

29a. foot-over-knee or

29b. seated rotation

31. hip flexor stretch

UPPER LEG

32a. seated hamstring stretch or

32b. lying hamstring stretch

34a. standing thigh stretch or

34b. kneeling thigh stretch

34c. kneeling two-legged stretch

LOWER LEG, ANKLE AND FOOT

39. top-of-toe stretch

Duration: 11 minutes

Golf

The body is used in an asymmetrical way, so ensure balance by stretching the active side and doing strength exercises for the other side. Back health is particularly important in this activity, since it involves so much rotation in the trunk.

ABDOMINALS

3a. standing side stretch or

3b. seated side stretch or

3c. kneeling side stretch

CHEST

4a. bent-arm wall stretch or

4b. doorway stretch or

4c. elbow squeeze

7. chest press

LOWER AND MIDDLE BACK

10. forward hanging stretch

11. lying torso twist

12a. frog stretch or

12b. standing pull-back

NECK

17. throat stretch

SHOULDERS

18. elbow up/elbow down

20. chicken

22a. kneeling hand clasp

22b. straight-arm bridge

FOREARM, WRIST AND HAND

27. hand press

HIPS

29a. foot-over-knee or

29b. seated rotation

31. hip flexor stretch

UPPER LEG

32a. seated hamstring stretch or

32b. lying hamstring stretch

34a. standing thigh stretch or

34b. kneeling thigh stretch or

34c. kneeling two-legged thigh stretch

LOWER LEG, ANKLE AND FOOT

37a. heel dip or

37b. double heel dip

Duration: 13 minutes 30 seconds

Hiking/backpacking

The action of walking extends the hip joint and so the hamstrings (and sometimes the gluteals) may tighten over time. If over-developed and inflexible, this can lead to lower back tightness and pain. If you are climbing hills or mountains, however, the calves will be employed significantly on the way up, and the thighs on the way down (by contracting they act as a braking system for the body), so these areas should be stretched.

CHEST

6. hand clasp

7. chest press

LOWER AND MIDDLE BACK

8. child pose

10. forward hanging stretch

12a. frog stretch or

12b. standing pull-back

UPPER BACK

13a. arm-across-chest

13b. hand-over-knee

14. snake

NECK

15. seated neck stretch

HIPS

28a. butterfly or

28b. squat stretch

29a. foot-over-knee or

29b. seated rotation

31. hip flexor stretch

UPPER LEG

32a. seated hamstring stretch or

32b. lying hamstring stretch

34a. standing thigh stretch or

34b. kneeling thigh stretch or

34c. kneeling two-legged thigh stretch

LOWER LEG, ANKLE AND FOOT

37a. heel dip or

37b. double heel dip

38. heel-down knee bend

41. outer ankle stretch

42. inner ankle stretch

Duration: 13 minutes

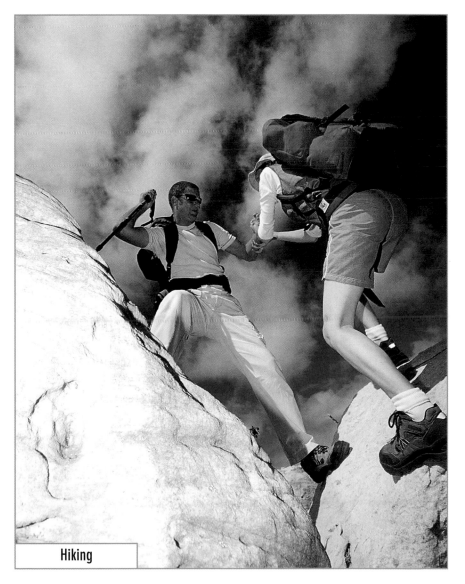

Hiking

Hockey

This sport also involves asymmetrical activity, so stretching the active side is important, while strengthening the other side. Pay particular attention to abdominals, obliques and the back.

ABDOMINALS

1a. cobra or

1b. kneeling back bend

3a. standing side stretch or

3b. seated side stretch

3c. kneeling side stretch

CHEST

6. hand clasp

LOWER AND MIDDLE BACK

10. forward hanging stretch

UPPER BACK

14. snake

FOREARM, WRIST AND HAND

27. hand press

HIPS

28a. butterfly or

28b. squat stretch

29a. foot-over-knee or

29b. seated rotation

30a. cross-legged lean forward or

30b. foot-on-knee

31. hip flexor stretch

UPPER LEG

32a. seated hamstring stretch or

32b. lying hamstring stretch

34a. standing thigh stretch or

34b. kneeling thigh stretch or

34c. kneeling two-legged thigh stretch

35a. seated stride or

35b. lying stride

LOWER LEG, ANKLE AND FOOT

37a. heel dip or

37b. double heel dip

38. heel-down knee bend

41. outer ankle stretch

42. inner ankle stretch

Duration: 13 minutes

Ice-skating/roller-blading

Since the action involves extension of the hip and the external rotation of the hip, it would follow that the hamstrings and the gluteals, particularly the gluteus maximus and the deep rotators of the hip, would need to be stretched in order to avoid tightness in these muscles.

ABDOMINALS

1a. cobra or

1b. kneeling back bend

3a. standing side stretch or

3b. seated side stretch or

3c. kneeling side stretch

LOWER AND MIDDLE BACK

10. forward hanging stretch

11. lying torso twist

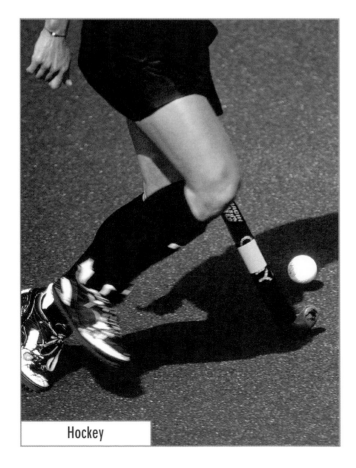

Hockey

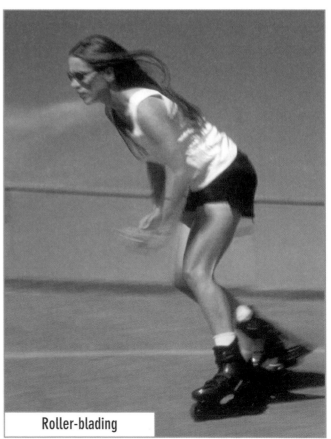

Roller-blading

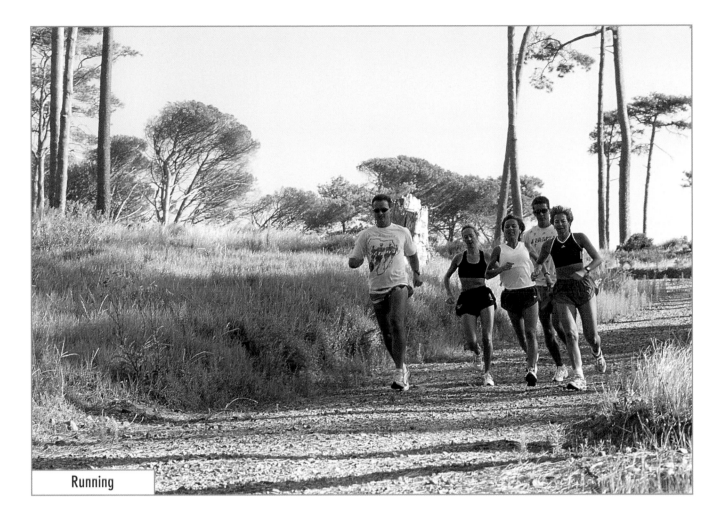

Running

NECK

16. lying neck stretch

HIPS

28a. butterfly

28b. squat stretch

29a. foot-over-knee or

29b. seated rotation

30a. Cross-legged lean forward

30b. foot-on-knee

31. hip flexor stretch

UPPER LEG

32a. seated hamstring stretch or

32b. lying hamstring stretch

34a. standing thigh stretch or

34b. kneeling thigh stretch or

34c. kneeling two-legged thigh stretch

35a. seated stride

35b. lying stride

36. ITB stretch

LOWER LEG, ANKLE AND FOOT

41. Outer ankle stretch

42. Inner ankle stretch

Duration: 12 minutes

Jogging/running

As in the case of hiking, running can lead to tightness in the calves, hamstrings and quadriceps.

ABDOMINALS

2. elevated back bend

3a. standing side stretch or

3b. seated side stretch or

3c. kneeling side stretch

CHEST

6. hand clasp

LOWER AND MIDDLE BACK

8. child pose

10. forward hanging stretch

HIPS

28a. butterfly

28b. squat stretch

29a. foot-over-knee or

29b. seated rotation

31. hip flexor stretch

UPPER LEG

32a. seated hamstring stretch or

32b. lying hamstring stretch

34a. standing thigh stretch or

34b. kneeling thigh stretch or

34c. kneeling two-legged thigh stretch

36. ITB stretch

LOWER LEG, ANKLE AND FOOT

37a. heel dip

38. heel-down knee bend

41. outer ankle stretch

42. inner ankle stretch

Duration: 12 minutes 30 seconds

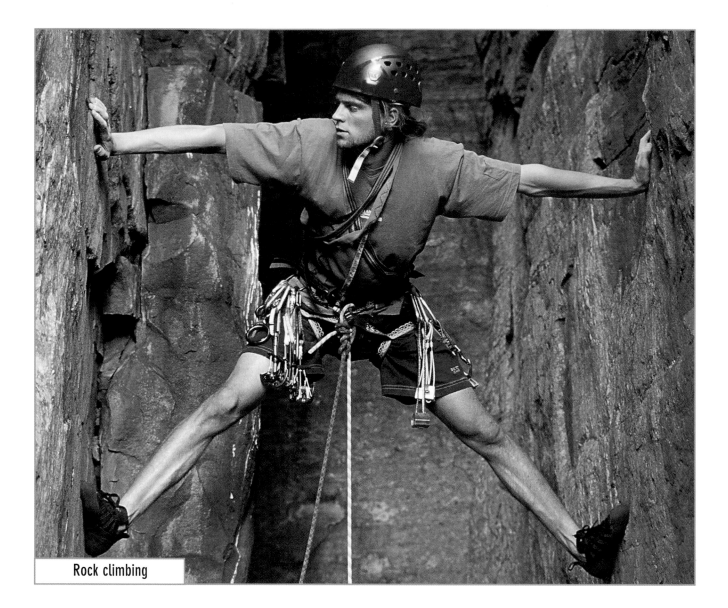

Rock climbing

Rock climbing

As with rowing, this is a sport that requires tremendous strength in the latissimus dorsi. So tightness in this muscle can be common, leading to possible lower back pain. It can also result in stiffness around the back of the shoulders and arms, which would hamper rock climbers when trying to grip overhead.

ABDOMINALS

1a. cobra or

1b. kneeling back bend

LOWER AND MIDDLE BACK

10. forward hanging stretch

12a. frog stretch or

12b. standing pull-back

UPPER BACK

13a. arm-across-chest or

13b. hand-over-knee

NECK

15. seated neck stretch

SHOULDERS

18. elbow up/elbow down

19. shoulder strap stretch

FOREARM, WRIST AND HAND

26. scarecrow stretch (with internal rotation)

27. hand press

HIPS

29a. foot-over-knee or

29b. seated rotation

30a. cross-legged lean forward or

30b. foot-on-knee

31. hip flexor stretch

UPPER LEG

33. downward dog stretch

34a. standing thigh stretch or

34b. kneeling thigh stretch or

35a. seated stride or

35b. lying stride

LOWER LEG, ANKLE AND FOOT

37a. heel dip or

37b. double heel dip

39. top-of-toe stretch

41. outer ankle stretch

42. inner ankle stretch

Duration: 13 minutes

Rugby/touch rugby/football

Much depends on the position you play, but in general you should keep your hamstrings and calves flexible, since these sports require much running.

ABDOMINALS

1a. cobra or

1b. kneeling back bend

3a. standing side stretch or

3b. seated side stretch

3c. kneeling side stretch

CHEST

4a. bent-arm wall stretch or

4b. doorway stretch or

4c elbow squeeze

LOWER AND MIDDLE BACK

10. forward hanging stretch

UPPER BACK

13a. arm-across-chest

13b. hand-over-knee

14. snake

NECK

15. seated neck stretch

SHOULDERS

18. elbow up/elbow down

HIPS

28a. butterfly or

28b. squat stretch

29a. foot-over-knee or

29b. seated rotation

31. hip flexor stretch

UPPER LEG

32a. seated hamstring stretch or

32b. lying hamstring stretch

34a. standing thigh stretch or

34b. kneeling thigh stretch or

34c. kneeling two-legged thigh stretch

35a. seated stride or

35b. lying stride

LOWER LEG, ANKLE AND FOOT

37a. heel dip or

37b. double heel dip

38. heel-down knee bend

41. outer ankle stretch

42. inner ankle stretch

Duration: 14 minutes

Scuba diving/snorkelling

The action of swimming underwater entails lying face down, while looking ahead, which puts the neck into excessive extension. This tends to compress that area of the spine which can lead to tension headaches. In extreme instances it can result in an imbalance of strength between the front and back neck muscles. This will lead to further postural problems as the rest of the body tries to compensate for the 'unnatural' position of the head on the neck.

ABDOMINALS

1a. cobra or

1b. kneeling back bend

LOWER AND MIDDLE BACK

8. child pose

10. forward hanging stretch

NECK

16. lying neck stretch

HIPS

29a. foot-over-knee or

29b. seated rotation

31. hip flexor stretch

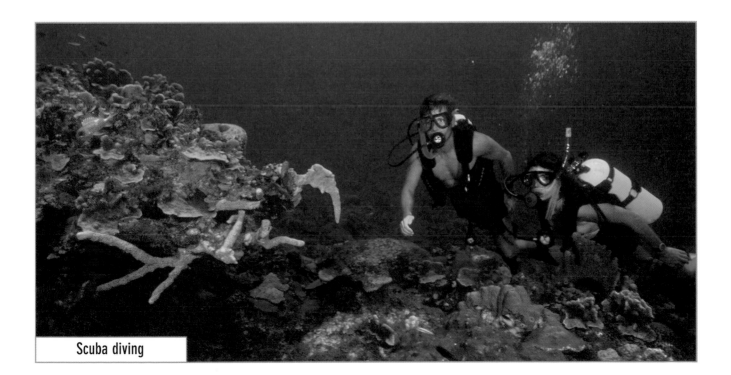

Scuba diving

UPPER LEG

32a. seated hamstring stretch or

32b. lying hamstring stretch

34a. standing thigh stretch or

34b. kneeling thigh stretch or

34c. kneeling two-legged thigh stretch

LOWER LEG, ANKLE AND FOOT

37a. heel dip or

37b. double heel dip

38. heel-down knee bend

40. bottom-of-toe stretch

Duration: 9 minutes

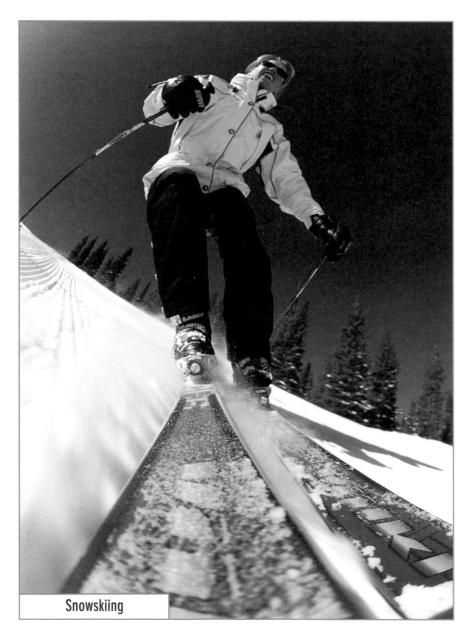

Snowskiing

Skiing

Concentrate on keeping the leg muscles and the lower back flexible.

ABDOMINALS

1a. cobra or

1b. kneeling back bend

CHEST

6. hand clasp

LOWER AND MIDDLE BACK

9. tree hug

10. forward hanging stretch

11. lying torso twist

12a. frog stretch

12b. standing pull-back

UPPER BACK

13a. arm-across-chest

13b. hand-over-knee

14. snake

SHOULDERS

18. elbow up/elbow down

19. shoulder strap stretch

FOREARM, WRIST AND HAND

27. hand press

HIPS

28a. butterfly or

28b. squat stretch

29a. foot-over-knee or

29b. seated rotation

30a. cross-legged lean forward or

30b. foot-on-knee

31. hip flexor stretch

UPPER LEG

32a. seated hamstring stretch or

32b. lying hamstring stretch

34a. standing thigh stretch or

34b. kneeling thigh stretch or

34c. kneeling two-legged thigh stretch

35a. seated stride

35b. lying stride

Duration: 13 minutes

Soccer/football

Keep the hamstrings, calves and quadriceps flexible and also the hip flexors of the 'striking' leg.

ABDOMINALS

1a. cobra or

1b. kneeling back bend

3a. standing side stretch or

3b. seated side stretch or

3c. kneeling side stretch

LOWER AND MIDDLE BACK

10. forward hanging stretch

11. lying torso twist

12b. standing pull-back

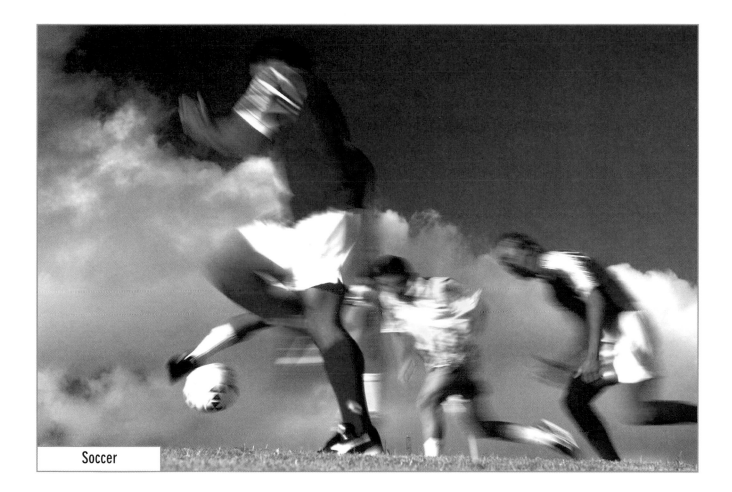

Soccer

NECK

15. seated neck stretch

HIPS

28a. butterfly or

28b. squat stretch

29a. foot-over-knee or

29b. seated rotation

30a. cross-legged lean forward or

30b. foot-on-knee

31. hip flexor stretch

UPPER LEG

32a. seated hamstring stretch or

32b. lying hamstring stretch

34a. standing thigh stretch or

34b. kneeling thigh stretch or

34c. kneeling two-legged thigh stretch

35a. seated stride or

35b. lying stride

LOWER LEG, ANKLE AND FOOT

37a. heel dip or

37b. double heel dip

38. heel-down knee bend

41. outer ankle stretch

42. inner ankle stretch

Duration: 14 minutes 30 seconds

Squash/tennis

Because people use only one arm when playing these sports, overuse injuries and problems arising from muscular imbalance are common. It is therefore important to stretch the 'active' side while also strengthening the under-used side.

ABDOMINALS

3a. standing side stretch or

3b. seated side stretch or

3c. kneeling side stretch

CHEST

4a. bent-arm wall stretch or

4b. doorway stretch or

4c. elbow squeeze

LOWER AND MIDDLE BACK

10. forward hanging stretch

UPPER BACK

13a. arm-across-chest

13b. hand-over-knee

SHOULDERS

18. elbow up/elbow down

20. chicken

FOREARM, WRIST AND HAND

25. kneeling wrist stretch (squash)

26. scarecrow stretch (with internal rotation, for squash)

27. hand press

HIPS

29a. foot-over-knee or

29b. seated rotation

31. hip flexor stretch

UPPER LEG

32a. seated hamstring stretch or

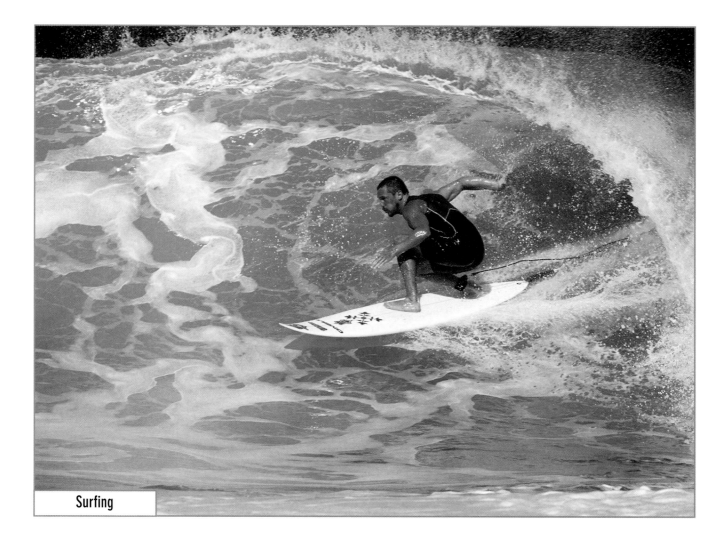

Surfing

32b. lying hamstring stretch

34a. standing thigh stretch or

34b. kneeling thigh stretch or

34c. kneeling two-legged thigh stretch

35a. seated stride or

35b. lying stride

LOWER LEG, ANKLE AND FOOT

37a. heel dip or

37b. double heel dip

41. outer ankle stretch

42. inner ankle stretch

Duration: 14 minutes (tennis routine) or 14 minutes 30 seconds (squash routine)

Surfing

When surfers paddle out to catch the waves, they assume a lying down posture, while looking up and forward. This can cause the same problems as those experienced by scuba divers. Surfers also tax their erector spinae, latissimus dorsi and the internal rotators of the arm (pectoralis major, subscapularis, teres major and deltoids). These need to be stretched well to avoid overuse injuries or imbalance issues.

ABDOMINALS

3a. standing side stretch or

3b. seated side stretch or

3c. kneeling side stretch

CHEST

4. bent-arm wall stretch or

4b. doorway stretch or

4c. elbow squeeze

LOWER AND MIDDLE BACK

8. child pose

10. forward hanging stretch

11. lying torso twist

12a. frog stretch or

12b. standing pull-back

UPPER BACK

13a. arm-across-chest or

13b. hand-over-knee

14. snake

NECK

16. lying neck stretch

SHOULDERS

18. elbow up/elbow down

19. shoulder strap stretch

UPPER LEG

32a. seated hamstring stretch or

32b. lying hamstring stretch

34a. standing thigh stretch or

34b. kneeling thigh stretch or

34c. kneeling two-legged thigh stretch

Duration: 10 minutes

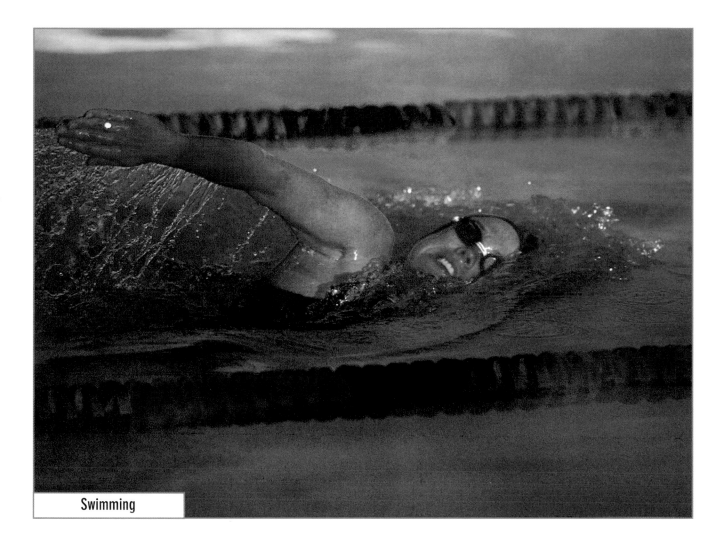

Swimming

Swimming/water polo

Keep the lower back and legs flexible. Muscles used in the upper back will depend on the stroke you use most. In water polo, watch out for tension in the lower back, abdominals and hips

ABDOMINALS

1a. cobra or

1b. kneeling back bend

CHEST

4. bent-arm wall stretch or

4b. doorway stretch or

4c. elbow squeeze

LOWER AND MIDDLE BACK

10. forward hanging stretch

12a. frog stretch or

12b. standing pull-back

UPPER BACK

13a. arm-across-chest

13b. hand-over-knee

14. snake

NECK

15. seated neck stretch

SHOULDERS

18. elbow up/elbow down

19. shoulder strap stretch

22a. kneeling hand clasp or

22b. straight-arm bridge

FOREARM, WRIST AND HAND

25. kneeling wrist stretch (water polo)

27. hand press (water polo)

HIPS

28a. butterfly or

28b. squat stretch

29a. foot-over-knee or

29b. seated rotation

31. hip flexor stretch

UPPER LEG

32a. seated hamstring stretch or

32b. lying hamstring stretch

34a. standing thigh stretch or

34b. kneeling thigh stretch or

34c. kneeling two-legged thigh stretch

35a. seated stride or

35b lying stride

LOWER LEG, ANKLE AND FOOT

37a. heel dip or

37b. double heel dip

Duration: 15 minutes (water polo),

13 minutes 30 seconds (swimming)

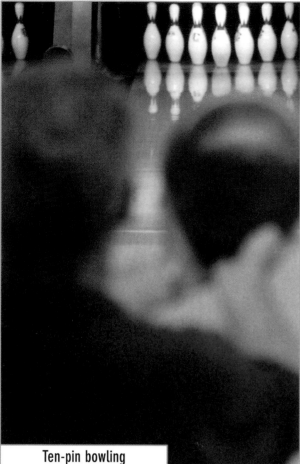

Ten-pin bowling

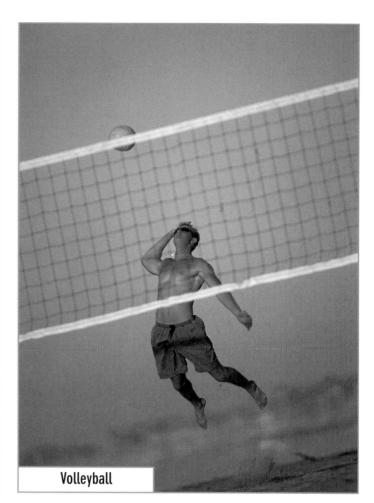

Volleyball

Ten-pin bowling/lawn bowls

Both these activities tend to make great demands on the shoulder muscles and the trunk will tend to rotate toward the side being used. As with any one-sided, asymmetric, activity, try to balance the body by stretching the side most used, while strengthening the opposite side.

CHEST

5. lying chest opener

LOWER AND MIDDLE BACK

9. tree hug

8. child pose

11. lying torso twist

UPPER BACK

13a. arm-across-chest or

13b. hand-over-knee

14. snake

SHOULDERS

18. elbow up/elbow down

19. shoulder strap stretch

UPPER ARM

23. straight-arm wall stretch

FOREARM, WRIST AND HAND

27. hand press

HIPS

29a. foot-over-knee or

29b. seated rotation

31. hip flexor stretch

UPPER LEG

32a. seated hamstring stretch or

32b. lying hamstring stretch

34a. standing thigh stretch or

34b. kneeling thigh stretch or

34c. kneeling two-legged thigh stretch

Duration: 10 minutes

Volleyball

There is a similarity to basketball in that the spine is put through various degrees of flexion and extension. There is also a fair amount of jumping. Keep the calves, hamstrings and lower back supple.

ABDOMINALS

1a. cobra or

1b. kneeling back bend

3a. standing side stretch or

3b. seated stretch or

3c. kneeling side stretch

CHEST

6. hand clasp

LOWER AND MIDDLE BACK

10. forward hanging stretch

12a. frog stretch

12b. standing pull-back

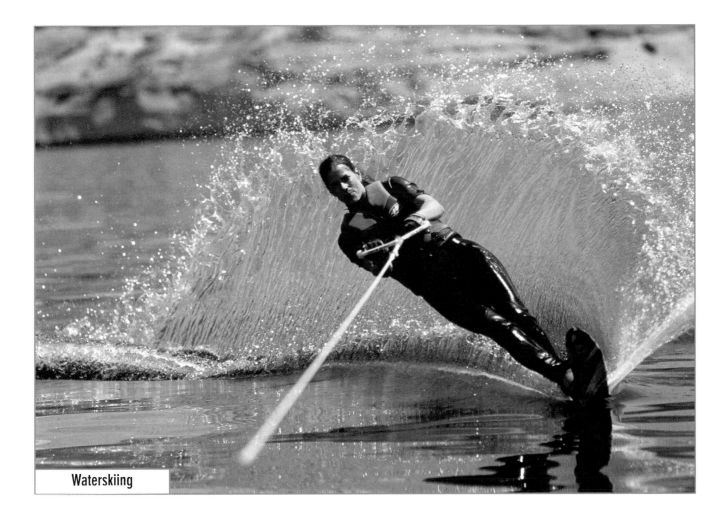

Waterskiing

UPPER BACK

14. snake

SHOULDERS

18. elbow up/elbow down

FOREARM, WRIST AND HAND

25. kneeling wrist stretch

26. scarecrow stretch (with internal rotation)

27. hand press

HIPS

30a. cross-legged lean forward or

30b. foot-on-knee

31. hip flexor stretch

UPPER LEG

32a. seated hamstring stretch or

32b. lying hamstring stretch

34a. standing thigh stretch or

34c. kneeling two-legged thigh stretch

35a. seated stride or

35b. lying stride

LOWER LEG, ANKLE AND FOOT

37a. heel dip or

37b. double heel dip

38. heel-down knee bend

41. outer ankle stretch

42. inner ankle stretch

Duration: 15 minutes

Waterskiing

The legs do most of the work. Due to a lean-back stance (not lean-forward as in snowskiing), concentrate on quadriceps and abdominals.

ABDOMINALS

1a. cobra or

1b. kneeling back bend

3a. standing side stretch or

3b. seated stretch or

3c. kneeling side stretch

3a. Standing side stretch or

3b. Kneeling side stretch (advanced)

LOWER AND MIDDLE BACK

10. forward hanging stretch

11. lying torso twist

12a. frog stretch or

12b. standing pull-back

UPPER BACK

13a. arm-across-chest or

13b. hand-over-knee

14. snake

SHOULDERS

18. elbow up/elbow down

22a. kneeling hand clasp or

22b. straight-arm bridge

UPPER ARM

23. straight-arm wall stretch

FOREARM, WRIST AND HAND

27. hand press

HIPS

29a. foot-over-knee

31. hip flexor stretch

UPPER LEG

32a. seated hamstring stretch or

32b. lying hamstring stretch

34a. standing thigh stretch or

34b. kneeling thigh stretch or

34c. kneeling two-legged thigh stretch

Duration: 11 minutes

Walking

The same muscles are used as for hiking, but on a lesser scale.

LOWER AND MIDDLE BACK

9. tree hug

10. forward hanging stretch

HIPS

28a. butterfly or

28b. squat stretch

29a. foot-over-knee or

29b. seated rotation

31. hip flexor stretch

UPPER LEG

32a. seated hamstring stretch or

32b. lying hamstring stretch

34a. standing thigh stretch or

34b. kneeling thigh stretch or

34c. kneeling two-legged thigh stretch

LOWER LEG, ANKLE AND FOOT

37a. heel dip or

37b. double heel dip

38. heel-down knee bend

Duration: 7 minutes 30 seconds

Windsurfing

The back muscles, specifically the lats, trapezius and rhomboids, are used extensively as well as the shoulders and biceps. Stretching these will help prevent a strong back-of-body overpowering a weak front-of-body.

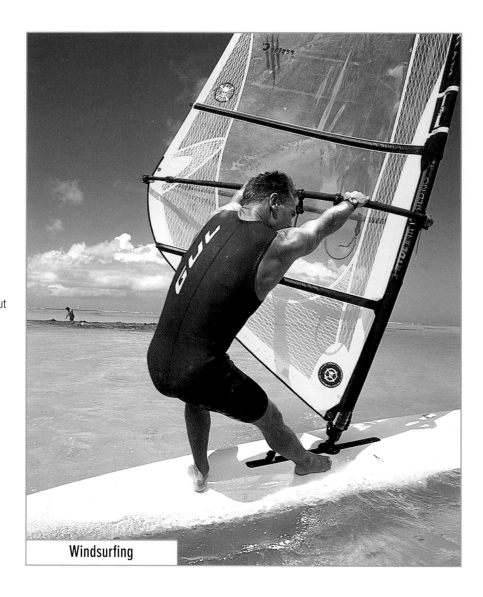

Windsurfing

ABDOMINALS

1a. cobra or

1b. kneeling back bend

3a. standing side stretch or

3b. seated side stretch or

3c. kneeling side stretch

LOWER AND MIDDLE BACK

8. child pose

11. lying torso twist

12a. frog stretch or

12b. standing pull-back

UPPER BACK

13a. arm-across-chest or

13b. hand-over-knee

NECK

15. seated neck stretch

SHOULDERS

18. elbow up/elbow down

19. shoulder strap stretch

UPPER ARM

23. straight-arm wall stretch

FOREARM, WRIST AND HAND

27. hand press

HIPS

31. hip flexor stretch

UPPER LEG

32a. seated hamstring stretch or

32b. lying hamstring stretch

34a. standing thigh stretch or

34b. kneeling thigh stretch or

34c. kneeling two-legged thigh stretch

Duration: 11 minutes 30 seconds

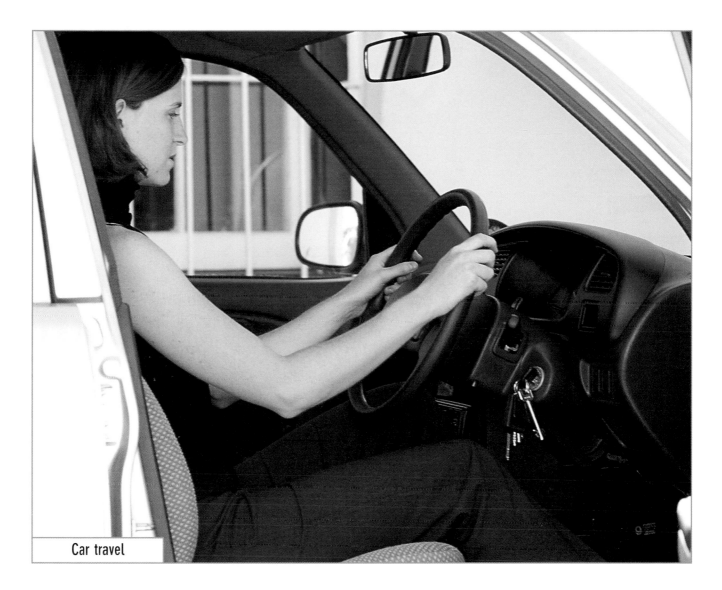

Car travel

LIFESTYLE STRETCHES

Air/car travel

Since air and car travel requires you to remain seated for long periods of time, you may want to look at doing more dynamic than static stretches. Mobilizing your muscles and joints will release built-up tension and assist circulation; refreshing and relaxing you in the process. Below are some modified mobilization stretches, combined with some relevant static stretches. You should be able to perform all these exercises while seated and with very little space to move.

ABDOMINALS

Mobilization

modified torso reach – seated

CHEST

Mobilization

modified chest opener – seated, with bent arms

LOWER AND MIDDLE BACK

Mobilization

modified cat stretch – seated

modified torso swing – seated, hands on lap

Stretches

10. modified forward hanging stretch – seated

12a. modified frog stretch – seated, with your hands up on the steering wheel (if you are in the driving seat) or the backrest of the chair in front of you if you are a passenger.

UPPER BACK

Mobilization

upper spine roll – seated

Stretches

14. snake – seated

NECK

Mobilization

head roll

Stretches

15. seated neck stretch

UPPER ARM

Mobilization

elbow bend

FOREARM, WRIST AND HAND

Mobilization

wrist roll

LOWER LEG, ANKLE AND FOOT

Mobilization

ankle roll

Gardening

Gardening involves a great deal of bending and kneeling and frequently you may hold these positions over long periods. Dynamic stretching will help release the tension and alleviate stiffness resulting from crouching in the same position for long. Below is a mix of mobilization and static stretches from which you can select a routine to suit you, depending on your gardening routine.

ABDOMINALS

Mobilization

torso reach

torso roll

Stretches

3a. standing side stretch or

3b. seated side stretch

3c. kneeling side stretch

CHEST

Mobilization

chest opener

Stretches

5. hand clasp

LOWER AND MIDDLE BACK

Mobilization

cat stretch

torso swing

Stretches

9. tree hug

10. forward hanging stretch

11. lying torso twist

UPPER BACK

Mobilization

upper spine roll

Stretches

14. snake

NECK

Mobilization

head roll

Stretches

16. lying neck stretch

SHOULDERS

Mobilization

arm swings

Stretches

18. elbow up/elbow down

FOREARM, WRIST AND HAND

Mobilization

wrist roll

Stretches

25. kneeling wrist stretch

26. scarecrow stretch

27. hand press

HIPS

Mobilization

hip roll or leg swing

Stretches

29a. foot-over-knee or

29b. seated rotation

31. hip flexor stretch

UPPER LEG

Mobilization

knee bend

Stretches

32a. seated hamstring stretch or

32b. lying hamstring stretch

34a. standing thigh stretch or

34b. kneeling thigh stretch or

34c. kneeling two-legged thigh stretch

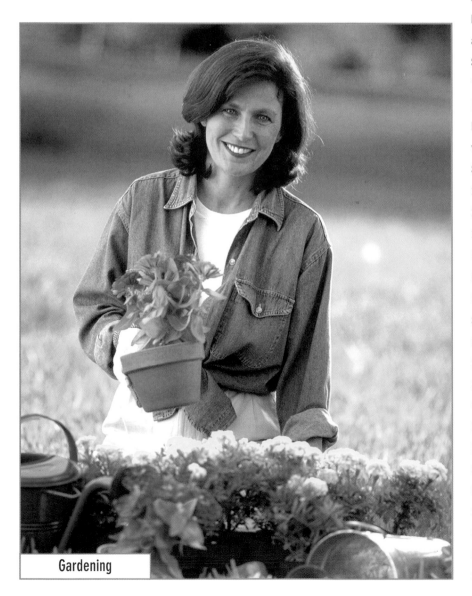

Gardening

Office/seated work

Office work usually involves sitting for most of the day, immobilizing your body over long periods. It follows then, that dynamic stretching will be most effective for releasing the tension in the muscles. Below are a mix of mobilization exercises and static stretches from which to select a routine to suit the time, space (and privacy) available to you at your work place.

ABDOMINALS

Mobilization

torso reach

torso roll

Stretches

3a. standing side stretch or

3b. seated side stretch

3c. kneeling side stretch

CHEST

Mobilization

chest opener

Stretches

7. chest press

LOWER AND MIDDLE BACK

Mobilization

cat stretch

torso swing

Stretches

8. child pose

9. tree hug

10. forward hanging stretch

11. lying torso twist

UPPER BACK

Mobilization

upper spine roll

Stretches

14. snake

NECK

Mobilization

head roll

Stretches

16. lying neck stretch

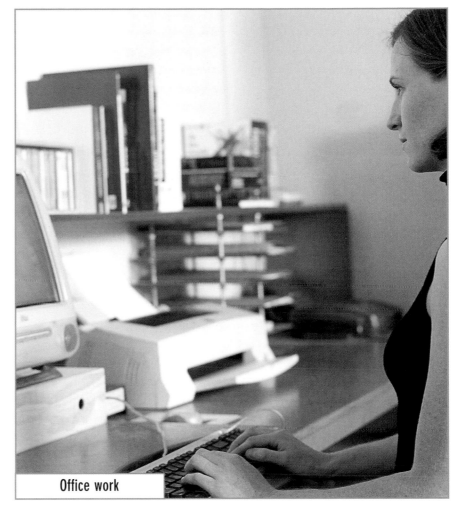

Office work

SHOULDERS

Mobilization

arm swings

Stretches

18. elbow up/elbow down

UPPER ARM

Mobilization

elbow bend

FOREARM, WRIST AND HAND

Mobilization

wrist roll

Stretches

25. kneeling wrist stretch

26. scarecrow stretch

HIPS

Mobilization

hip roll

leg swing

Stretches

29a. foot-over-knee or

29b. seated rotation

30a. cross-legged lean forward

31. hip flexor stretch

UPPER LEG

Mobilization

knee bend

gentle leg swing

Stretches

32a. seated hamstring stretch or

32b. lying hamstring stretch

34a. standing thigh stretch or

34b. kneeling thigh stretch or

34c. kneeling two-legged thigh stretch

LOWER LEG AND ANKLE

Mobilization

ankle roll

Glossary

Abduction: Movement of a limb away from the centreline of the body, such as lifting a straight arm laterally from one's side.

Adduction: Movement of a limb toward the centreline of the body, such as pulling a straight arm toward one's side.

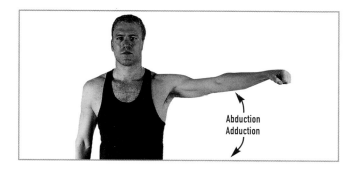

Abduction
Adduction

Aerobic exercise (with oxygen): Activity in which the body is able to supply adequate oxygen to the working muscles for a period of time, e.g. running or cycling.

Agonist: The primary muscle that contracts in order to create a specific movement.

Anaerobic Exercise, (without oxygen): Activities in which oxygen demands of muscles are so high that they rely upon an internal metabolic process for oxygen. Short bursts of 'all-out' activities such as sprinting or weightlifting are anaerobic.

Antagonist: The muscle that works in cooperation with the agonist muscle and can move the joint in the opposite way to the movement caused by the agonist.

Anterior: The front side.

Ballistic stretch: A more vigorous stretch, using a swinging or bouncing motion suited only for conditioned athletes (often used in martial arts and dancing).

Cardiovascular training: Physical conditioning that strengthens the heart and blood vessels, the result of which is an increase in the ability of the muscles to use fuel more effectively.

Cervical spine: The seven vertebrae of the neck.

Cool-down: Rhythmic, low-intensity aerobic activities that provide a transition period between high-intensity aerobic work and less aerobically taxing activities.

Cross-training: Engaging in a variety of physical activities and exercise modalities including cardiovascular and strength training exercises. A training method used to help minimize boredom, maintain motivation and prevent overuse syndrome.

Depression: Pulling down the shoulders. The movement is opposite to shrugging or pulling shoulders up under the ears.

Dynamic flexibility: The ability to use the muscles to move the joint through its range of motion.

Electrolytes: Elements capable of conducting electricity in solution. Examples are potassium, sodium and chloride.

Endurance: Ability to sustain a physical activity or to continue exerting a force over time.

Extension: Extending a joint, or opening the angle between two bones; straightening out.

External rotation: The outward or lateral rotation of a joint within the transverse plane of the body. The movement will be towards the posterior (back) surface of the body.

Flexibility: A joint's ability to move freely through the full range of motion (ROM) allowed by its structure. This may involve movement in one plane only (hinge joints such as the knee), or movement in all directions (ball and socket joints such as the hip and shoulder). In order to achieve and maintain a joint's ROM, it is necessary to stretch the muscles that move those joints.

Flexion: Flexing a joint or closing the angle between two bones.

Hyperextension: The extension of a joint beyond the natural anatomical position.

Inferior: To be below, lower, or at the bottom.

Intensity: Degree of resistance, energy required or degree of difficulty as related to a workout.

Internal rotation: The inward or medial rotation of a joint within the transverse plane of the body. Movement is directed toward the anterior (front) surface of the body.

Ischiopubic ramus (sitting bones): The flattened inferior projection of the hipbone below the obturator foramen consisting of the united inferior rami of the pubis and ischium.

Kyphosis: An increased concavity of the thoracic curve of the spine.

Lateral: To the side.

Lats: The latissimus dorsi or upper back muscles.

Ligament: Strong, fibrous band of connecting tissue connecting two or more bones or cartilage or supporting a muscle, fascia or organ.

Lordosis: Increased concavity of the lumbar curve of the spine (hollow back).

Lumbar: The five vertebrae of the lower back.

Multijoint: Actively involving more than one joint.

Muscle tone: A term referring to firm muscles.

Overload: Training harder than one is used to.

Overload principle: Applying a greater load than normal to a muscle in order to increase its capability.

Pecs: The pectoralis or chest muscles.

Performance benefit: Improvement in physical fitness or strength as a result of exercise.

Plyometric exercise: Where muscles are loaded suddenly and stretched, then quickly contracted to produce a movement. Athletes who must jump do these, i.e. jumping off bench to ground, quickly rebounding to another bench.

Posterior: Located behind a part or toward the rear of the body.

Primary movement: The main movement around a specific joint.

Pronation: The internal rotation of the foot or forearm.

Prone position: Lying on the stomach.

Quads: The quadricep muscle group.

Rom: (Range of Motion) The amount of movement at each joint. Every joint in the body has a 'normal' range of motion. Joints maintain their normal range of motion by being moved.

Sagittal plane: A division that separates the body into a left and right half. Movements in the sagittal plane are in the forward-backward direction.

Scoliosis: Sideward curvature of the spine.

Sitting bones (ischiopubic ramus): The flattened inferior projection of the hipbone below the obturator foramen consisting of the united inferior rami of the pubis and ischium.

Static flexibility: The ability to assume an extended position and then hold it still.

Superior: Above, on top of or upper.

Supination: The external rotation of the foot or forearm.

Supine: Lying on the back.

Tendon: A band of strong, fibrous tissue that connects muscle to the bone.

Thoracic: The 12 vertebrae of the mid-spine.

Transverse plane: The division separating the body into an upper and lower half. Movements are in the horizontal direction or parallel to the ground.

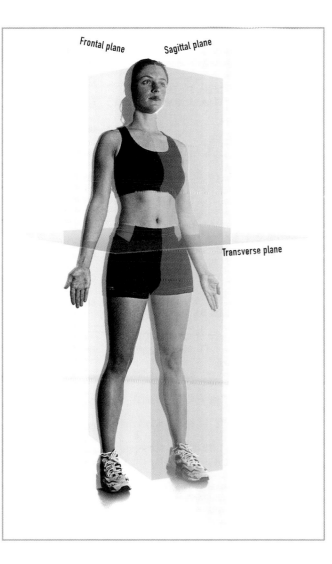

Warm-up: A balanced combination of increasingly intense aerobic exercises that prepare the body and the mind for more vigorous exercise.

Further Reading

Belling, N. (2003). *The Yoga Handbook*. London: New Holland Publishers

Briffa, J. (2002). *Ultimate Health*. London: Penguin Group

Cochram, S. and House, T. (2000). *Stronger Arms and Upper Body*. Champaign, IL, USA: Human Kinetics

Complete Guide to the Human Body. (2002). Noble Park, Victoria, Australia: The Five Mile Press

Energise Your Life. (2001). London: Duncan Baird Publishers

Graham, H. (2002). *The Lazy Man's Guide to Exercise*. Dublin: New Leaf

Green, B. (2002). *Get with the Program*. New York: Simon & Schuster

Holford, P. (1997). *Optimum Nutrition Bible*. London: Piatkus

Holford, P. (1998). *100% Health*. London: Piatkus

Human Body Atlas. (2002). Willoughby, Australia: Grange Books

Lamond, P. (2002). *Pilates*. London: New Holland Publishers

Malcolm, L. (2001). *Health Style*. London: Duncan Baird Publishers

New Atlas of Human Anatomy. (1999). London: Constable

Urla, J. (2002). *Yogilates*. London: Thorsons

Websites

www.fitnesszone.co.za

An excellent site. Loads of information covering all aspects of health, fitness and nutrition. Allows you to pose questions to a fitness expert. Books and videos are also on offer.

www.acefitness.org

Another good site covering all aspects of health, nutrition and fitness. Although it deals more with the education of fitness practitioners, it also provides an enormous amount of information that will be of interest to the layman.

www.anatomical.com

Charts relating to anatomy, training heart rates, weight training illustrations, alternative health therapies, health education, etc. Videos and books also available.

www.ciavideo.com

Videos of workouts by various presenters in the United States – great for exercising at home.

www.musclemedia.com

Specifics regarding weight-training issues. Back orders of magazines are also available, as well as information on nutrition specific to weight training.

www.sportsci.org

Although this is a very scientific site, there are some good articles on research relating to various sports and the issues affecting them, such as hydration, training, nutrition, etc.

www.turnstep.com

Good for ordering exercise videos. Some articles of interest are included, but are more for instructors.

www.ideafit.com

Although mainly aimed at fitness instructors and trainers, this site includes articles the layperson may find interesting and valuable – go to 'publications'.

www.topendsports.com/testing/

This site relates specifically to fitness testing. Tests range from very scientific to home-based and easy to use. Also lists various fitness-related books.

http://primusweb.com/fitnesspartner/index.html

Lists various fitness-related sites and relevant articles.

www.dolfzine.com

Extensive range of articles covering diverse issues such as training, nutrition, dieting, exercise during pregnancy, yoga, Pilates, how to choose a personal trainer, among others.

http://groups.yahoo.com/group/Supertraining/

This site is devoted to sports, strength and fitness science, as well as training, therapy and education. You will need to join the group in order to access the information posted.

www.fitpro.com

Primarily aimed at fitness practitioners, but has some good articles for the layperson, covering a wide range of health and fitness-related topics.

Photographic Credits

Copyright rests with the following photographers and/or their agents listed below. Key to Locations: t = top l = left; r = right.
(No abbreviation is given for pages with a single image, or pages on which all photographs are by the same photographer.)

GI = galloimages/gettyimages.com   PA = Photo Access   MF = Masterfile SA   SIL = Struik Image Library

Cover		GI	86		Burazin/MF	106 l & r	PA
6–7		Miguel Salmmeron/MF	93		Miguel Salmeron/MF	107	Ryno/SIL
8		GI	95, 96		Nicholas Aldridge/SIL	108	Clinton Waits/SIL
9–11		PA	98		Peter Griffith/MF	109–115	PA
21	l	Cecconi/SIL	99–101		PA	116	Simon Bornhoft/SIL
21	r	Ryno/SIL	102		Michael Cowell/SIL	117	Ryno/SIL
22		PA	103		PA	118	PA
23	t	Allen Birnbach/MF	104		Michael NG/SIL	119	Ryno/SIL
38		PA	105		Jacques Marais/SIL		

Acknowledgements

AUTHOR'S DEDICATION
To Stu, with love

AUTHOR'S ACKNOWLEDGEMENTS
Many thanks to my editor Anna Tanneberger, designer Geraldine Cupido, photographer *extraordinaire* Danie Nel and everyone else who helped behind the scenes at NHP. Thanks to commissioning editor Alfred LeMaitre for his support. Thanks also to my gorgeous models – Paul, Vanessa, Clint, Joon and Nikki and dear friends and colleagues Mark Vella (for his sharp eye and tireless commitment) and Sally Lee (for her willing and expert advice). Lastly – many, many thanks and a great deal of love to mom, dad, Marls, Jax and Sprog – my very large and very special family, who mean the world to me.

PUBLISHER'S ACKNOWLEDGEMENTS
The Publisher would like to thank the models; The Nike Concept Shop at the Victoria & Alfred Waterfront, Cape Town for supplying the clothing; Chrysna for the styling; and Mark Vella for overseeing the shoot.